6/13/96 Rec. from
Steve Fowles

Property of ~~Steve Fowles~~ phil Jacklin

DHEA
A PRACTICAL GUIDE

Ray Sahelian, M.D.

DHEA: A Practical Guide

Published by Be Happier Press
PO Box 12619
Marina Del Rey, CA 90295
310-821-2409

Printed in the United States of America
Desktop Publishing by TMS/Russell Kurtz, Ph.D.,
    russtms@earthlink.net

Sahelian, Ray
    DHEA: a practical guide/ Ray Sahelian, M. D.
    p.cm.
    Includes bibliographical references and index.
    ISBN 09639755-8-7
    Library of Congress Catalog Card Number 96-84272

    1. Dehydroepiandrosterone I. Title
    QP572.A3S34 1996   615'.364   QB196-20361

Warning– Disclaimer

Acknowledgements

I wish to sincerely thank the following researchers and clinicians for taking time out of their busy schedules to share their knowledge and experience.

Researchers

Elizabeth Barrett-Connor, M.D., Department of Family and Preventive Medicine, University of California, San Diego, in La Jolla, CA.

Etienne-Emile Baulieu, M.D., Ph.D., Professor, College of France, Paris, and Director of the Institut National de la Sante et de la Recherche Medicale (similar to the US NIH), Department of Hormone Research.

Michael Bennett, M.D., Department of Pathology, University of Texas Southwestern Medical Center in Dallas.

John Buster, M.D., Director, Division of Reproductive Endocrinology and Infertility, Department of Obstetrics and Gynecology, Baylor College of Medicine, Houston, TX.

David Herrington, M.D., Division of Cardiology, The Bowman Gray School of Medicine, Winston-Salem, NC.

Christopher Heward, Ph.D., Endocrinologist and Research Director, Emerald Laboratories, Carlsbad, CA.

Peter Hornsby, Ph.D., Huffington Center on Aging, Baylor College of Medicine, Houston, TX.

Elias Ilyia, Ph.D., Clinical and Research Director, Diagnostechs Laboratory, Seattle, WA.

Robert Jesse, Ph.D., M.D., Director of the Acute Cardiac Care Program, Medical College of Virginia, Richmond.

Seymour Lieberman, Ph.D., St. Luke's-Roosevelt Hospital Center, New York, NY.

Marc Lane, Ph.D., Gerontological Research Center, National Institute on Aging, Baltimore, MD.

Christopher Longcope, Ph.D., Department of Obstetrics and Gynecology, University of Massachusetts Medical School, Worcester.

Maria Majewska, Ph.D., National Institute on Drug Abuse, Medications Development Division, Rockville, MD.

Joseph Mortola, M.D., Department of Reproductive Endocrinology, Beth Israel Hospital and Harvard Medical School, Boston, MA.

M. S. Rao, M.D., Department of Pathology, Northwestern University Medical School, Chicago, IL.

Arthur Schwartz, Ph.D., Fels Institute for Cancer Research and Molecular Biology, Temple University School of Medicine, Philadelphia, PA.

Ron von Vollenhoven, M.D., Ph.D., Division of Immunology and Rheumatology, Stanford University Medical Center, CA.

Roy Walford, M.D., Professor, University of California Los Angeles, co-author, along with Lisa Walford, *The Anti-Aging Plan* (Four Walls Eight Windows).

Owen Wolkowitz, M.D., Department of Psychiatry, University of California, San Francisco.

Clinicians

Eric Braverman, M.D., Director of Path Medical/Path Foundation, Princeton, NJ.

Edmund Chein, M.D., Director of Palm Springs Life Extension Institute, CA.

Ward Dean, M.D., Medical Director of The Center for Bio-Gerontology in Pensacola, FL, and author of *Biological Aging Measurement – Clinical Applications* (Center for Bio-Gerontology, 1988).

Arnold Fox, M.D., author of *Alternative Healing*, Beverly Hills, CA.

Alan Gaby, M.D., author of *Preventing and Reversing Osteoporosis* (Prima Publishing, Rocklin, CA), Past President of the American Holistic Medical Association, Editor of *Nutrition and Healing* newsletter.

Allen Green, M.D., Medical Director, Institute for Holistic Treatment and Research, Newport Beach, CA.

Dale Guyer, M.D., Saint Vincent's Hospital, Department of Complementary Medicine, Indianapolis, IN.

Ron Hoffman, M.D., New York City, NY; Program Chairman of the American College for the Advancement of Medicine.

Douglas Hunt, M.D., private practice, Burbank, CA.

Michael Janson, M.D., Barnstable, MA, President Elect of American College for Advancement in Medicine; author, *The Vitamin Revolution in Health Care* (Arcadia Press, 1996).

Richard Kunin, M.D., San Francisco, CA, President of the Society for Orthomolecular Health-Medicine.

Davis Lamson, N.D., Private Practice, Tahoma Clinic, Kent, WA.

Lord Lee-Benner, MD, Private Practice, Newport Beach, CA.

Christian Renna, D.O., Private Practice, Dallas, TX.

Gary Ross, M.D., Private Practice, San Francisco, CA.

David Schechter, M.D., Clinical Faculty, University of Southern California, Department of Family Medicine, and private practice, West Los Angeles, CA.

Gerald Sugarman, M.D., Director of Lifetime Wellness in Arroyo Grande, CA.

Murray Susser, M.D., Author of *Solving the Puzzle of Chronic Fatigue Syndrome*, Santa Monica, CA.

Karlis Ullis, M.D., Assistant Clinical Professor, University of California, Los Angeles, and Director, Sports Medicine Preventive Group, Santa Monica, CA.

Jonathan V. Wright, M.D., Tahoma Clinic, Kent, WA. Editor of *Nutrition and Healing* newsletter, and bestselling author of *Healing with Nutrition*.

A special "thank you" to **Steven Wm. Fowkes,** Executive Director of the Cognitive Enhancement Research Institute, Menlo Park, CA, for his assistance with this manuscript. Mr. Fowkes is also the publisher of an interesting newsletter called *Smart Drug News*, tel. 415-321-CERI.

ABOUT THE AUTHOR

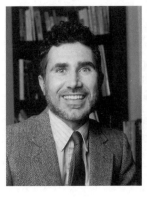 **Ray Sahelian, M.D.,** is a physician certified by the American Board of Family Practice. He obtained a Bachelor of Science degree in nutrition from Drexel University and completed his doctoral training at Thomas Jefferson Medical School, both in Philadelphia. Following graduation he worked for three years as a resident in family medicine at Montgomery Hospital in Norristown, PA, and was involved with all aspects of medical care including pediatrics, cardiology, obstetrics, oncology, psychiatry, and surgery.

A popular and respected physician and medical writer, Dr. Sahelian is internationally recognized as a moderate voice in the evaluation of leading-edge nutrients and hormones. He has been seen on numerous television programs including *CNN Talk Live, The Maury Pauvich Show, A Current Affair, Extra, Dini Petty Show* (Canada), and *Zone Interdite* (France); mentioned by countless major magazines such as *Newsweek, US News and World Report, Cosmopolitan, Modern Medicine, Health,* and *Internal Medicine News;* and quoted in hundreds of newspapers including *USA Today, The Los Angeles Times, The Washington Post, The Miami Herald, The Denver Post, Le Monde* (France), and *Que Pasa* (Chile). His articles have appeared in *Let's Live, Total Health, Healthy and Natural,* and others. Millions of listeners from over 1,000 radio stations nationwide have heard him discuss the latest research on hormones and nutrients.

Dr. Sahelian is the Editor-In-Chief of *Melatonin, DHEA, and Longevity Update,* and a nationally-known lecturer. He is also the author of the highly acclaimed *Be Happier Starting Now* and the bestselling *Melatonin: Nature's Sleeping Pill.*

AUTHOR'S NOTE

Over the next few months and years you will come across many opinions on DHEA. There will be enthusiasts who will claim it as the "fountain of youth," while others may warn you not to take it at all. The media will have many stories and articles about this hormone, both pro and con. A controversy will brew and continue for a long time and chances are you will be totally confused and not know whose opinion to follow.

I've sifted through hundreds of articles on DHEA, from the 1950s to the very latest research, and interviewed prominent researchers and physicians who have studied and prescribed this hormone.

My goal is to provide you with an informed opinion discussing the benefits of DHEA, its uncertainties, and its shortcomings. I will provide you the information, and then it will be up to you, in consultation with your health care professional, to decide whether DHEA is appropriate for your unique circumstance.

Please keep in mind that although there are a large number of studies evaluating the role of DHEA in laboratory animals, the research with humans is limited.

Ray Sahelian, M.D.

Contents

INTRODUCTION

Will it someday be possible to take a hormone pill on a daily basis and live longer? Most of you probably trust that science will eventually discover such a pill. What about now? Is there a hormone some people are currently taking that is known to prolong life?

Did you shake your head *No*? Think again... Are you still shaking your head *No*?

Why do doctors prescribe the hormone estrogen to women after menopause? Not to purposely shorten their life span! There is a sharp decline in estrogen levels after menopause, which often occurs in most women in their late 40s. A study whose results were published in the *American Journal of Public Health* in 1995 evaluated the connection of estrogen replacement therapy (ERT) with death and illness in over 40,000 postmenopausal women followed for 6 years. Compared with women who never used hormone replacement therapy, current users had a lower rate of heart disease, colon cancer, and hip fracture. On the other hand, there was a higher rate of endometrial cancer and a slightly higher rate of breast cancer. Overall, though, women on ERT lived longer.

Another study done by Dr. Bruce Ettinger at the Kaiser Permanente Medical Care Program in Oakland, CA, and published in the January 1996 issue of the journal *Obstetrics and Gynecology*, showed that women who supplement estrogen after menopause live longer than women who don't. Most of the benefits come from a reduction in heart disease.

So there's preliminary evidence to support that at least one hormone, estrogen, when replaced, can help women live longer after menopause. There's still some debate on which form, dosage, or combination, of estrogens (estrone, estradiol, estriol, or Premarin [horse estrogens]) will provide the best benefits with the fewest risks. There's also evidence to suggest that when estrogen is combined with progesterone, the risk of endometrial cancers will decline. Based on the two studies mentioned above, and the numerous other studies on ERT that have already been published over the past two decades, most doctors recommend postmenopausal women start ERT. These doctors do not realize that they are practicing anti-aging medicine.

What about DHEA and all the other hormones that decline with aging? Should we replace them all? Science cannot yet give us definitive answers. However, we do ourselves a favor by keeping an open mind to the possibility that, in the future, at least some additional hormone supplements may help us be healthier, happier, and more youthful much longer than we ever expected; and maybe allow us to stroll in the park while holding the tiny hand of our great-great-great-grand-child.

References:

Ettinger B, Friedman GD, Bush T, Quesenberry CP Jr. *Reduced mortality associated with long-term postmenopausal estrogen therapy*. Obstet Gynecol 87:6-12, 1996.

Folsom AR, Mink PJ, Sellers TA, Hong CP, Zheng W, Potter JD. *Hormonal replacement therapy and morbidity and mortality in a prospective study of postmenopausal women*. Am J Public Health 85:1128-32, 1995.

Grady D, Rugin S, Petitti D. *Hormone therapy to prevent disease and prolong life in postmenopausal women*. Ann Intern Med 117:1016-37, 1992.

ONE

THE ABCs OF DHEA

Controversy is not new to the health food and supplement industry. In 1995, melatonin, a hormone made by the pineal gland, generated a lot of discussion, became big news, and even got its own cover on the November 6th issue of *Newsweek*. Now DHEA seems to be gradually taking a brighter spotlight, especially since it has become readily available without a prescription. We now have two hormones over-the-counter easily purchased and used (or misused) by the consumer.

If you thought claims about melatonin were hyped, confusing, and controversial... If you thought everybody you asked had a different opinion about its benefits and shortcomings... Just wait and see what researchers and doctors are saying about DHEA.

What does DHEA stand for?

DHEA is short for dehydroepiandrosterone (D-hi-dro-epp-E-an-dro-stehr-own), a *hormone* made by the adrenal glands located just above the kidneys (see figures). All words in italics are defined in the glossary.

Is DHEA a new hormone that we've discovered?

Scientists have known about this hormone since 1934 and there have been thousands of articles published about it since then. However, only a small percentage of these studies have involved human subjects.

Why all the hype about DHEA?

Back in 1994, researchers at the University of California, San Diego, School of Medicine, wanted to find out what would happen to older individuals if they got supplements of DHEA (Morales and Yen). We'll discuss this study more fully in the next chapter.

The researchers gave middle-aged volunteers 50 mg of DHEA nightly for 3 months. There was an increase in physical and psychological well-being. The subjects reported enhanced energy, deeper sleep, improved mood, more relaxed feelings, and an improved ability to deal with stressful situations.

When the results of this study were published, there was a flurry of publicity. Stories about DHEA appeared in newspapers and magazines. Radio and television picked it up. Eventually, many national TV shows did a segment on it. However, since DHEA was not easily available to the consumer, it didn't become popular as quickly as melatonin did.

One of the reasons that this study caused so much publicity was that it was supported by many dozens of previous studies, most conducted in rodents, that indicated DHEA to have a benefit in heart disease, cancer, diabetes, weight loss, lupus, and a variety of other conditions. Some people started calling DHEA "the fountain of youth."

Before the Morales and Yen study was published, DHEA was already well known in the holistic health community. Articles about this steroid had appeared in many alternative magazines and newsletters.

Is DHEA safe?

Whenever doctors talk about the safety of a medicine they separate it into short-term safety over a few days or weeks, and long-term safety over months and years of use. Dr. Nestler, a researcher at the Medical College of Virginia/Virginia Commonwealth University in Richmond, has given 1600 mg of DHEA a day for 4 weeks to healthy young men without any serious side effects (Nestler, 1988). At this dosage there was a lowering of cholesterol and a decrease in body fat, with a greater response in obese individuals. Most DHEA supplements on the market are less than 50 mg.

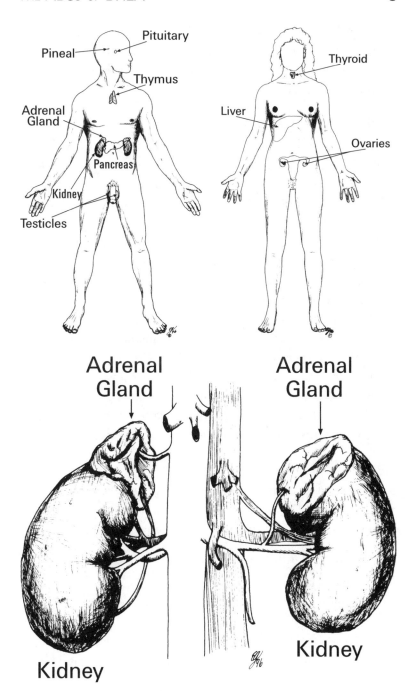

Pituitary

Pineal

Thymus

Adrenal
Gland

Pancreas

Kidney

Testicles

Thyroid

Liver

Ovaries

Adrenal
Gland

Adrenal
Gland

Kidney

Kidney

As to the safety of using DHEA for 5, 10, 20 years or longer, no formal human studies have been published; then again, few long-term human studies have been done for any medicines, hormones, or nutrients.

Is DHEA the only adrenal hormone?

More than 150 hormones are known to be synthesized by the adrenal glands. However, the most abundant hormone made by the adrenal glands is DHEA. We'll discuss the adrenal glands–with a diagram of DHEA's chemical synthesis and *metabolism*–in more detail in Appendix A.

After DHEA is made by these glands it goes into the blood-stream, and from then on it travels all over the body and goes into our cells, where it is converted into male hormones, known as *androgens,* or female hormones, known as *estrogens* (Drucker, 1972). Whether DHEA gets converted predominantly into andro-gens or estrogens depends on a person's medical condition, age, and sex. Every person has a unique biochemistry.

In males the testicles also make androgens, while in females, before menopause, the ovaries also make estrogens. So the body has developed at least two organs where sex steroids are made. After menopause, the ovaries no longer make estrogens.

How much DHEA does our body make?

It is estimated that humans make between 10 and 15 mg of DHEA and DHEAS a day (Longcope, 1995), although estimates have been up to 25 mg. This number may be lower for women.

How is DHEAS different from DHEA?

When DHEA is metabolized, a chemical called sulfate is added. Sulfate consists of the mineral sulfur combined with oxygen (SO_4). Thus DHEAS stands for DHEA-sulfate.

DHEA is mostly made in the morning hours. Its levels decline fairly rapidly during the day because it is quickly cleared by the kidneys. However, DHEAS is cleared much more slowly and blood levels remain much more stable throughout the day (Longcope, 1995). About 90% of this steroid in the blood is in the DHEAS form; the rest circulates as DHEA. That is why, when researchers want to assess blood levels for DHEA, they often measure DHEAS levels.

When you take DHEA supplements, some will circulate in your bloodstream as DHEA, but most of it will be sulfated by your liver to circulate as DHEAS.

Will taking DHEA supplements suppress my adrenal gland's natural DHEA production?

The production of most steroids is controlled by a "feedback loop," which means that when hormone levels get too high, the body is told to make less, and when the hormone levels are too low, the body is told to make more. *Cortisol, testosterone,* and estrogen are all regulated by this feedback. In other words, if you take cortisol, or a similar derivative such as prednisone, it will shut off your body's natural production.

Fortunately, DHEA appears to be one of the exceptions. According to Dr. Peter Hornsby at the Baylor College School of Medicine in Houston, TX, there doesn't seem to be a feedback mechanism for DHEA or DHEAS. In other words, supplements are not likely to stop our body's own production, although there are no long-term human studies to confirm this.

Where does the DHEA that I buy come from?

The DHEA pills that you buy are made by vitamin and pharmaceutical companies. They extract sterols from wild yams, the most common sterol being *diosgenin*. After cleaving a few side chains from diosgenin in the laboratory, DHEA is produced.

Will natural yam extract pills increase my DHEA levels?

Most of the DHEA sold now is synthetic DHEA. However, some vitamin companies do sell extracts of wild yams in pill form.

Some even promote these yam-extract products as "DHEA precursor complexes" or "natural DHEA."

To get to the bottom of the yam-extract conversion issue, I asked a leading expert in the field, Seymour Lieberman, Ph.D., from St. Luke's-Roosevelt Hospital Center, New York, NY, who has been studying DHEA (which he calls 'dehydro') and other steroids longer than most researchers in the field (55 years so far!). He is one of the top experts in the world on the biochemical aspects of DHEA.

Congratulations on publishing such a detailed and thorough article on the metabolism of DHEA and other steroids in the *Annals of the New York Academy of Sciences*.

Thank you. Dehydro is my favorite topic. It's a fascinating compound and we only know a fraction of what we need to know.

Some vitamin stores sell wild yam extracts. There are claims that these yams have compounds which can be converted into DHEA by the body. Is this possible?

DHEA is made commercially from a plant of the Dioscorea *family* [wild yams] *found in abundance in Mexico. Extracts of this plant contain a steroidal saponin which may be converted in a laboratory by a series of 6 to 8 chemical reactions into DHEA. A comparable series of reactions is not known to exist in nature and certainly not in humans.*

Consequently it is highly unlikely, perhaps impossible is a better word, that the ingestion of extracts of the Dioscorea *plant will lead to the formation, by metabolic transformation of the relevant plant constituent, to either pregnenolone or DHEA.*

In a word, Dr. Lieberman means "No."

Do animals also make DHEA?

Significant amounts of DHEA are made only by humans and primates, such as apes, gorillas, and monkeys. Rodents, such as mice or rats, have only small amounts circulating in their bloodstream. DHEA administration in rodents has often shown beneficial effects. But many researchers caution about making health claims for humans based on rodent studies.

What can I do to keep my DHEA(S) level up?

Leading a relaxed lifestyle with high psychological well-being (easier said than done) can help you live longer and maintain optimal DHEAS levels. Stress can decrease DHEAS levels (Labbate, 1995). As to the role of exercise, one study did not find an association. Ninety-six patients with coronary artery disease were started on an exercise program and had their DHEAS levels measured. After 12 weeks, there was no change in the levels of this hormone (Milani, 1995). The researchers conclude, "Although behavior therapy in combination with exercise training was previously shown to lead to increase in DHEAS, exercise training alone has no significant impact on DHEAS, thereby strengthening the suggested role of behavioral changes in modifying this hormone."

Is it okay if I self-medicate with DHEA?

I recommend that you see a health care practitioner who is familiar with its use before taking this hormone.

What if my doctor is not knowledgeable about DHEA?

Unfortunately, most doctors at this time are not familiar with DHEA therapy. I had a telephone conversation with a colleague from residency, Lou Mancano, M.D., who is now the co-director of the Family Practice Residency Program at Montgomery Hospital in Norristown, Pennsylvania. Because he is involved in a teaching hospital supervising residents, Dr. Mancano keeps up with the latest standard medical research. His account is probably typical of most doctors:

I practice traditional medicine, in a traditional hospital, and I am familiar with DHEA, but only in the context of checking levels in women who present to the office with hirsutism (excess hair) and uncontrolled acne. Basically, the reason for checking DHEA levels is to find out if there is an adrenal tumor that accounts for the excess. When the DHEA levels are very high, I order a CAT scan of the abdomen, and if an adrenal tumor is found, I refer the patient to a surgeon.

I didn't know that this steroid was available without a prescription. I also didn't know that DHEA levels decline with age until now that you told me. I religiously read all the medical journals that are sent to doctors, and I don't remember seeing any articles on DHEA.

It wouldn't surprise me if the majority of physicians in the country also are not aware that DHEA levels decline with age. I've never thought of this steroid in terms of a deficiency state, but always in terms of excess.

The concept that DHEA can be used as hormone replacement therapy either by itself or with estrogen and other hormones is intriguing. Keep me in touch with your latest findings.

If you can't find a physician in your area who is familiar with the use of DHEA, see the last page of this book.

A personal story

Martin is 64 years old. In the summer of 1995 he read in a major news magazine a discussion of the study done by Drs. Morales and Yen at the University of California, San Diego. He immediately phoned his doctor to ask if he could start on DHEA. His doctor said, "What's that?"

After a number of phone calls, and a great deal of persistence, Martin found a doctor who not only had heard of DHEA, but had been prescribing it to his patients for 3 years. Martin's blood levels showed him to be low in this hormone compared to a young person. He was started on 20 mg a day.

I spoke to Martin in April of 1996. He was introduced to me by a friend. He had been on DHEA for 6 months. I asked him if he had been helped by this supplement.

After about a month of taking it, I noticed that my energy level was higher, and I was more relaxed.

Anything else?

Yes. There's been a remarkable influence on my sexual satisfaction. My libido has improved, and I feel 30 years younger when I'm intimate with someone.

(While thinking to myself that perhaps I should give it a try, even though I'm only 38...) Any side effects?

None so far. I've had blood levels drawn which show my levels are back to those in the young. Martin paused... *Doctor, there's something I want to ask you. You've studied this hormone a great deal... Do you think I could live longer if I keep taking it?*

References:

Drucker MD, Blumberg JM, Gandy HM, David RR, Verde AL. *Biologic activity of DHEAS in man.* J Clin Endocrinol Metab 35:48-54, 1972.

Hornsby P. *Biosynthesis of DHEAS by the human adrenal cortex and its age-related decline.* Ann NY Acad Sci 774:29-46, 1995.

Labbate L, Fava M, Oleshansky M, Zoltec J, Littman A, Harg P. *Physical fitness and perceived stress. Relationships with coronary artery disease.* Psychosomatics 36(6): 555-60, 1995.

Longcope C. *Metabolism of DHEA.* Ann NY Acad Sci 774:143-148, 1995. "DHEA circulates in a nonproteinated form and it is bound weakly to sex hormone-binding globulin and albumin. DHEAS is strongly bound to albumin and also undergoes reabsorption from renal tubules accounting for its higher levels and longer duration in serum than DHEA."

Milani R, Lavie C, Barbee R, Littman A. *Lack of effect of exercise training on DHEAS.* Am J Med Sci 310(6):242-6, 1995.

Morales A, Nolan J, Nelson J, Yen S. *Effects of replacement dose of DHEA in men and women of advancing age.* J Clin Endocrinol Metab 78:1360-7, 1994.

Nestler J, Barlascini C, Clore J, Blackard W. *DHEA reduces serum low density lipoprotein levels and body fat but does not alter insulin sensitivity in normal men.* J Clin Endocrinol Metab 66:57-61, 1988.

TWO

Happy 120ᵗʰ Birthday??

Not all of the hormones produced in our bodies decline with aging. Estrogen, made by the ovaries, declines dramatically only after menopause. Melatonin, made by the pineal gland, declines progressively as the decades march on. DHEA and DHEAS, made by the adrenal glands, also progressively drop with aging starting in our late 20s. However, other steroids made by the adrenal glands, such as *cortisol* and *aldosterone*, stay relatively stable throughout life. Furthermore, the amount of androgens produced by the testicles drops only slightly with aging.

A number of changes occurs in our bodies as we age. There's a substantial reduction in protein synthesis leading to shrinkage in muscle mass, and decreased bone formation leading to osteoporosis. Many researchers think that these changes are closely related to the age-associated decline in hormones. Some even think that restoring these declining hormones could 1) delay muscle wasting, 2) strengthen bones, 3) maintain a healthy heart, and 4) slow the progression of aging. I will discuss the connections between hormone replacement therapy and life extension in the rest of this chapter.

From infancy to 120– DHEA throughout life

The pattern of DHEA(S) production by the human body is interesting. Although a fetus makes DHEA(S), and this hormone is present in a baby for the first few months of life, there is very little made from 6 months up to the beginnings of puberty. From then on the levels continually rise, and peak in our 20s. From our 30s on, there is a progressive decline in DHEA(S) levels

(Orentreich, 1984). It is estimated that by age 70 we only make a fourth of the amounts made in our prime, and by age 90, perhaps a tenth (Migeon, 1957; Birkenhager-Gillesse, 1994; Ravaglia, 1996).

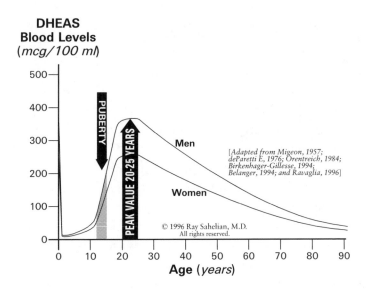

Please note that this graph is only an average based on limited studies. There are certain healthy older individuals who have higher blood levels of this steroid than their younger counterparts.

Since DHEA is the precursor to androgens and estrogens, the decline in DHEA production also reflects itself in the cells of our bodies. It is thought that at least half of the androgen and estrogen precursors in our body comes from the adrenal glands' DHEA. The rest are made in the testicles and ovaries.

After menopause, when the ovaries are practically no longer functioning, 100% of the estrogen precursors comes from the adrenal glands' DHEA (Labrie, 1991).

From mice to men, and women

Most of the longevity studies showing increased life span with DHEA have been done on rodents (Lucas, 1985). Although the majority of these studies confirm a life span extending effect with DHEA, we should keep in mind that, unlike humans, rodents have little circulating DHEA(S) in their blood (Nestler, 1995). This, alone, should caution us about jumping to conclusions based on results of animal studies. Dr. Peter Hornsby, from Baylor College of Medicine in Houston, TX, emphasized this when he wrote, "Although experiments in rodents on the effects of DHEA have been extremely valuable, we should always bear in mind the difficulty in applying rodent data to humans... In rodents, tissues may respond to DHEA quite differently since they do not normally have high levels of DHEA in their plasma."

Countless rodent studies with DHEA have shown increased life span and positive influences on a variety of illnesses such as heart disease, diabetes, and cancer. I have purposely chosen not to focus on these studies because conclusions from animal findings extrapolated to humans can sometimes be misleading and inaccurate. As much as possible, human studies have been emphasized in this book.

A group of human volunteers gets DHEA

Drs. Morales, Nelson, Nolan, and Yen, from the Department of Reproductive Medicine, University of California, San Diego, School of Medicine, wanted to find out the influence of DHEA supplements on middle-aged and older individuals. (I briefly mentioned this 1994 study in Chapter 1.) They were aware that aging is associated with a gradual shift from a 'young' state characterized by the building-up of muscles and tissues, called anabolism, to an 'aged' state characterized by the loss of muscle mass and strength, called catabolism.

These researchers recruited 13 men and 17 women who ranged from 40 to 70 years of age. Using a randomized, placebo-controlled, cross-over trial, they provided 50 mg of DHEA nightly for 3 months. During the study period they measured blood levels of many hormones and nutrients including androgens, lipids, and *insulin*, as well as body fat, *libido*, and sense of well-being. Within two weeks of treatment, the DHEAS levels in the bloodstreams of those receiving supplements reached those found in young adults.

A striking finding became apparent. The researchers state: "DHEA supplementation resulted in a remarkable increase in perceived physical and psychological well-being for both men and women. The subjects reported increased energy, deeper sleep, improved mood, more relaxed feelings, and an improved ability to deal with stressful situations."

Interestingly, no changes were noted in libido or body fat. Changes in blood lipids levels such as *cholesterol* were not significant. We'll discuss DHEA and libido in the next chapter.

Based mostly on results of this relatively short-term study, a number of people started DHEA supplements and a lot of media hype was generated. Articles appeared in various newspapers and magazines. Even *Newsweek's* August 7, 1995, article on melatonin had a sidebar titled, "DHEA: Nature's Other Time-Stopper?"

In order to find out whether higher doses and a longer period of treatment would have a more significant effect, Drs. Yen, Morales, and Khorram (1995) gave 100 mg of DHEA to 8 men and 8 women between the ages of 50 and 65 for 6 months– twice the dose and twice as long as the earlier study.

With 100 mg of DHEA on board, the serum levels of DHEAS increased several-fold in both men and women. The androgen levels doubled in the men, and quadrupled in the women. One of the eight women developed facial hair that resolved by the end of the study.

There were many biological markers assessed throughout the study. Lean body mass showed an increase in both genders, there was some increase in muscle strength of the knee, and no change was found in lipid profiles, insulin or glucose levels, nitrogen balance, bone mineral density, or basal metabolic rate. Interestingly, there was no mention of DHEA's effect on well-being as had been reported in the earlier study of 3 months.

Here are some theoretical mechanisms on how supplemental DHEA can increase life span, remembering, though, that as of yet there is no proof that it does so in humans:

- Improving immunity
- Turning on "youth" genes in our DNA that may be shut off by low levels of DHEA in old age
- Decreasing the rate of heart disease by lowering cholesterol and acting as a blood thinner
- Decreasing the rate of cancer
- Improving insulin's function thus better regulating blood sugar levels
- Balancing DHEA/cortisol ratios. As we age DHEA levels drop but cortisol levels stay relatively the same. This unbalanced ratio may have harmful consequences on blood sugar and immunity, among others
- Inhibition of glucose-6-phosphate dehydrogenase enzyme. This enzyme is involved in cancer promotion, lipid formation, and production of toxic oxygen free radicals

Do DHEA supplements have a role in hormone replacement therapy and can they influence longevity?

I asked the world's top researchers for their opinions:

Elizabeth Barrett-Connor, M.D., Department of Family and Preventive Medicine, University of California, San Diego, in La Jolla.

There is no evidence DHEA or DHEAS is good for women, except for a weak association with bone density. It may be good for men, but clinical trials are needed– as in large, randomized, double blind studies. None are yet available.

Michael Bennett, M.D., from the Department of Pathology at the University of Texas, Southwestern Medical Center in Dallas, has been researching DHEA's effects on the immune system.

DHEA does not have the bad effects that androgenic steroids, such as those used by some body builders, have. It is a precursor to estrogen which can possibly lead to breast enlargement in men if used in high doses. In women, high doses could pose the risk of an overabundance in androgens leading to such side effects as hirsutism (excess body hair). Many strains of mice have lived longer when supplemented with this steroid.

I'm 60 years of age. If my blood test showed that my level was low, I would consider taking low doses such as 25 mg to bring my levels higher. However, I would prefer being part of an experiment to test the effects of low-dose DHEA.

Etienne-Emile Baulieu, M.D., Ph.D., Director of the Institut National de la Sante et de la Recherche Medicale, Department of Hormone Research, Paris, France.

This is my favorite theory. We are studying the possible beneficial effects of re-establishing a "young" level of DHEAS in people over 60 years of age. The comparison to estrogen replacement therapy after menopause is a good one.

However, we need long-term studies to make sure that there are no negative effects on hormone-responsive tumors such as prostate and breast. We are currently doing studies on DHEA's role in cerebral function, cardiovascular system, bones, muscles, skin, metabolic (lipids, glucose), and hormonal (pituitary, insulin) parameters. We expect important influences by DHEA on most of these functions.

I would consider taking 25 mg or 50 mg daily if my blood levels were found to be low.

Peter J. Hornsby, Ph.D., from the Huffington Center on Aging, Baylor College of Medicine in Houston, TX, is an expert on the biosynthetic aspects of DHEA.

We have to do some long-term human experiments. The longest one published is 6 months. That's not long enough for us to know what would happen if we took it for 10 or 20 years. Our knowledge about DHEA is basically what it was a couple of decades ago with estrogen. Even after 20 years or so of research on estrogen, we still don't know its full effects.

Moreover, we really can't extrapolate from rodents to humans, because rodents have very low circulating DHEA(S) levels. Although they do make it, they do so locally in the brain and in gonadal tissues. When DHEA is given to rodents, any dose is basically a pharmacological dose [unnaturally high], *not a physiological dose.*

When asked "What cautions would you like to have mentioned in a book on DHEA?"

Don't take it except as part of a controlled clinical trial.

Maria Majewska, Ph.D., Medications Development Division, National Institute on Drug Abuse, Rockville, MD.

While we are waiting for more data (Dr. Baulieu's group is doing clinical studies at this time in France), the existing evidence already suggests that DHEA(S) replacement may be a safe and effective means of improving health and the quality of life during aging. However, we have yet to learn the right dosages.

John Nestler, M.D., Division of Endocrinology and Metabolism, Medical College of Virginia/Virginia Commonwealth University, Richmond (as reported in the *Annals NY Acad Sci* 774: ix-xi, 1995).

The clinical issues that will have to be addressed include optimal DHEA dosage, form and amount, route of administration, and delineation of side effect profile. It is important that such studies be conducted before DHEA is casually administered to men and women, as some physicians in private practice are currently doing, because DHEA administration may be associ-

ated with some untoward effects. For example, DHEA can be converted to potent androgens, such as testosterone, which would masculinize women. Similarly, whether DHEA administration is associated with any change in prostatic volume or risk for prostatic cancer in men is currently unknown.

Although the results of human DHEA studies appear promising and tantalizing, they still need to be confirmed in large-scale and properly controlled studies. Nonetheless, given the current groundswell in human DHEA-related research, I remain confident that these issues will be fully addressed within the next 5 to 10 years and predict that a therapeutic role for DHEA will be established. This could take the form of hormone replacement therapy (for example, starting DHEA administration around age 30 and keeping the serum level at its peak) or pharmacologic therapy for specific disease indications.

Seymour Lieberman, Ph.D., St. Luke's-Roosevelt Hospital Center, New York, NY.

The evidence thus far is so suggestive that it warrants further investigation.

Christopher Longcope, Ph.D., Department of Obstetrics and Gynecology, University of Massachusetts Medical School, Worcester.

Supplementing with DHEA will not do much. You might just as well take sugar pills. I doubt if DHEA will help people live longer.

Joseph Mortola, M.D., Department of Reproductive Endocrinology, Beth Israel Hospital and Harvard Medical School, Boston, MA.

I definitely think this hormone should be considered for replacement therapy, at least in the future, and perhaps now. DHEA has different effects on men and women, therefore, the recommendations and cautions would be different for each sex.

DHEA administration can have an estrogenic effect in tissues of women. I'm only speculating, but if women are on estrogen replacement therapy and they want to add DHEA, they can probably decrease the estrogen dose by half. Even though metabolites of DHEA will stimulate breast tissue, they will do so less than estrogen itself, thus possibly decreasing the risk of breast tumor initiation that has been suggested by some studies on estrogen replacement.

There has been speculation that testosterone, as well, may be appropriate for some women as replacement therapy. Since DHEA also gets converted into testosterone and other androgens in postmenopausal women, it may be a better way to deliver testosterone to tissues. However, lipid profiles and glucose levels should be monitored in women on DHEA.

In men, DHEA should be considered as having more estrogenic effects rather than androgenic. DHEA has some effects by binding to androgen receptors located everywhere through our bodies. This would, in men, act as a buffer to the effects of testosterone. The data are clear that DHEA is beneficial in men, and certainly can't hurt. But, the dosages have not been worked out.

Based on everything I know, I would take DHEA if I were older. I'm 42 now. Perhaps in my fifties I would start supplementing, but, by then, I would have the luxury of knowing the results of another decade of studies. As to older people not wanting to wait that long, I can see a justification for them using it now, as long as they are monitored by a qualified physician.

Arthur Schwartz, Ph.D., from Fels Institute for Cancer Research and Molecular Biology, Temple University School of Medicine in Philadelphia, PA, has been studying the role of DHEA in protecting against cancer.

I can understand people not wanting to wait for the unequivocal clinical data since it will take us years and years before we have any. Many of them are going to be dead before then. Some legitimately may want to take the risk, and I can't argue with that. If people want to do it, so be it. My own feeling is that 25 or 50 mg is not dangerous, but it's not going to do much, either. The chances for these low dosages to influence aging are zilch.

The dramatic effects on rodents in treating or preventing diabetes, cancer, and heart disease are usually achieved at high doses, and if we extrapolate these dosages from rodents to humans, it would be somewhere near 1,000 mg per day or higher, much higher than the 50 mg per day that people are using to supplement with. Perhaps humans don't need as much, but we don't know. However, at these high dosages, the androgenic effects of DHEA may be unacceptable.

Owen Wolkowitz, M.D., from the Department of Psychiatry at the University of California, San Francisco, has been studying DHEA for the last seven years. His focus recently has been on the role of this steroid in mood and memory.

There's a huge possibility. This hormone could potentially offer beneficial effects just as estrogen does, although the specific benefits need to be worked out.

I would not recommend doctors use DHEA replacement therapy at this time outside of the context of a research trial, partly because of medico-legal reasons, and partly because we don't know the long-term consequences.

When asked, "What about the argument that if we were to wait, we would have to wait decades to find the answers?"

That's true. I still think it's better to be cautious. Medicine's dictum is "first do no harm." But, personally, I may use this steroid on myself, if, in my later years, I find that I'm not as energetic as I used to be and there are no medical conditions to account for it. If my DHEA levels were low, I would consider taking it for a few weeks to see what it did. If there were benefits, I would continue. However, if I had no symptoms, even if my levels were low, I wouldn't see any reason to take DHEA.

Drs. Yen, Morales, and Khorram, Department of Reproductive Medicine, University of California, San Diego (as reported in *Ann NY Acad Sci* 774:128-142, 1995).

DHEA in appropriate replacement doses appears to have remedial effects with respect to its ability to induce an anabolic growth factor, increase muscle strength and lean body mass, activate immune function, and enhance quality of life in aging men and women, with no significant side effects. Further studies are needed.

Do you think DHEA has a role in hormone replacement therapy in older adults?

I asked this question of several clinicians who have been using DHEA in their practices.

Edmund Chein, M.D., a physician who practices anti-aging medicine in Palm Springs, CA, has used DHEA with several hundred patients.

I have not noticed any effect of DHEA on muscle mass or weight loss when a person has been placed on physiologic replacement dosages. I don't treat with DHEA, I use it, along with other hormones such as pregnenolone, growth hormone, progesterone, and testosterone, to replace low levels of hormones back up to youthful numbers. They all work together and a balance is crucial.

When asked, "Is DHEA the 'fountain of youth?'"

Of course not. No study on this planet has shown that it reverses any of the biomarkers of aging such as skin turgor, aerobic capacity, cell regeneration, and so on. If anything can be called the "fountain of youth," it's growth hormone.

Arnold Fox, M.D., is a physician in Beverly Hills, CA, and the co-author, along with Barry Fox, Ph.D., of *Alternative Healing* (Career Press). He has treated close to 200 patients with DHEA.

Yes. Yes. I take it. My wife takes it.

Most men and women have low DHEA levels after age 50.

At the initial exam I do a complete blood test and give them articles on DHEA. On the second visit, I discuss the results with them, and if their blood level is low we make a combined decision on whether to start replacement therapy with this hormone. I recite to my patients Cicero, the Roman philosopher's, words, "Old age must be resisted and its deficiencies restored."

Ward Dean, M.D., Medical Director of The Center for Bio-Gerontology in Pensacola, Florida and co-author of *Smart Drugs and Nutrients* and *Smart Drugs II.*

I've treated about 30 patients with DHEA. This steroid is absolutely appropriate for hormone replacement therapy. I start my patients in their 40s, and at a dose of 25 mg taken in the morning. DHEA is highest in the morning and giving it at that time would follow the normal circadian rhythm. The studies in mice that showed improvement in a variety of biochemical and physiological factors with DHEA supplementation encourage me to use this steroid.

Generally I don't do blood tests since they are expensive and the results are inconsistent. Based on a number of human studies, we know that the levels decline with aging.

Alan Gaby, M.D., is the author of *Preventing and Reversing Osteoporosis* (Prima, 1994), Past President of the American Holistic Medical Association, and a leading expert on nutrition.

DHEA, without a doubt, has a role to play in hormone replacement therapy. I have treated at least 300 patients and find this steroid to be helpful for anti-aging purposes as far as increasing muscle strength, better density of bone, and improved skin color. It's hard to say whether wrinkles have improved.

Gary Ross, M.D., in practice for 18 years in San Francisco, CA, has treated at least 200 individuals with DHEA.

Replacement therapy with this hormone should be considered for almost everyone in their late 30s and older if their blood levels are low. I have people on DHEA as young as 37. The longest that I've treated a person is 3 years.

Karlis Ullis, M.D., Assistant Clinical Professor, University of California, Los Angeles, and Director, Sports Medicine Preventive Group, Santa Monica, CA.

I think DHEA has anti-aging potentials, but therapy has to be individualized. There are some individuals who may benefit, while others would not. Our knowledge of this hormone is still too early; we're going to need a lot more studies.

And now, my opinion (I've stayed quiet so far, but I absolutely can't hold my peace any longer)

As indicated in this chapter, the consequences of human supplementation with DHEA for anti-aging purposes is, at this time, not fully known. The early research promises many benefits; then again, there may be some totally unexpected negative long-term effects. No number of studies on rodents will give us any definite clues to what will happen in humans since, among many other differences in metabolism, rodents have little DHEA(S) circulating in their blood.

Therefore I recommend you be skeptical of anyone who tries to convince you to take megadoses of this hormone because his pet mouse has been on it, does nonstop jumping jacks all day long, and has outlived (and outbred) all the other mice in the neighborhood.

Even given the beneficial effects that have been reported, we don't know whether the ideal dosage is 100 mg, 50 mg, 10 mg, or 5 mg. Is it better to supplement once daily, twice, or three times? Does the timing of the dosage make a difference, *i.e.*, morning or evening? Will men respond more favorably than women, or vice versa? Is bringing DHEA levels back to those of "youth" really the best strategy, or is it better to raise your DHEA levels into the upper half of the normal range for your age?

Having presented these uncertainties, I do not rule out the possibility that there could be an anti-aging role for DHEA supplementation in middle-aged and older individuals. Many early studies show promise. Hormone replacement therapy will continue being one of the most researched, and controversial, topics in health and medicine over the next few years, and even decades.

Now that estrogen/progesterone replacement therapy for women has gained a great deal of acceptance, the controversy has shifted to men. Should aging men take replacement testosterone to be healthier and happier? And let's not ignore the question of whether women should take replacement dosages of testosterone as well. Although a lot of people may not realize it, women make testosterone and men make estrogen. It's a matter of emphasis. In women, estrogens are dominant over androgens, and in men, androgens are dominant over estrogens. Both sexes make both hormones under normal, healthy circumstances.

Without a doubt, patients will be continuously asking their doctors whether they should supplement not only with DHEA, but with melatonin, growth hormone, progesterone, testosterone, estrogen, thyroid hormones, and others. The uncertainties and controversies will continue for a very long time.

If you are planning to supplement with DHEA, the very least I can recommend is that you make every effort to be supervised by a physician who is familiar with the research and has some amount of clinical experience with this steroid.

Martin ponders...

I was hoping you'd give me a more definite answer, but I appreciate your frankness that we still know very little about this hormone. Okay, so there is hope, but no guarantee, that this steroid is going to help me live longer. But what about the sense of well-being and sexual enjoyment that I've had since starting this steroid... Are these just placebo effects?

References:

Belanger A, Candas B, Dupont A, Cusan L, Diamond P, Gomez JL, Labrie F. *Changes in serum concentrations of conjugated and unconjugated steroids in 40 to 80 year old men.* J Clin End Met 79:1086-1090, 1994. "The small decrease in the serum concentrations of progesterone and pregnenolone in the presence of increased levels of cortisol and markedly decreased levels of DHEA and its polar metabolites suggests that adrenal 17, 20-lyase is particularly affected by aging."

An important point to keep in mind is that even though levels of DHEA(S) decline significantly with aging, their metabolites decrease to a smaller extent. This indicates that there is compensation going on in our cells to make up for the declining blood levels.

This study found a 60% decrease in DHEA and DHEAS between ages of 40 and 80.

Birkenhager-Gillesse E, Derksen J, Lagaay A. *DHEAS in the oldest old, aged 85 and over.* Ann NY Acad Sci 719: 543-52, 1994.

de Peretti E, Forest M. *Unconjugated DHEA plasma levels in normal subjects from birth to adolescence in humans.* J Clin Endocrinol Metab 43:982-90, 1976.

de Peretti E, Forest MG. *Pattern of plasma DHEAS levels in humans from birth to adulthood: evidence for testicular production.* J Clin Endocrinol Metab 47(3):572-7, 1978.

Hornsby P. *Current challenges for DHEA research.* Ann NY Acad Sci 774: xiii-xiv, 1995.

Labrie F. *Intracrinology.* Mol Cell Endocrinol 78:C113-C118, 1991.

Lucas J, Ahmed SA, Casey LM, MacDonald PC. *Prevention of autoantibody formation and prolonged survival in New Zealand Black/New Zealand White F1 mice fed DHEA.* J Clin Invest 75:2091-3, 1985.

Majewska M. *Neuronal actions of DHEA: Possible roles in brain development, aging, memory, and affect.* Ann NY Acad Sci 774:111-120, 1995.

Migeon C, Keller A, Lawrence. *DHEA and androsterone levels in human placenta. Effect of age and sex: day-to-day and diurnal variations.* J Clin End Met 17:1051-1062, 1957.

Morales A, Nolan J, Nelson J, Yen S. *Effects of replacement dose of DHEA in men and women of advancing age.* J Clin Endocrinol Metab 78:1360-7, 1994. DHEA levels reached those of young adults within 2 weeks of therapy. In women, a 2-fold increase in serum levels was noted for androgens such as testosterone, dihydrotestosterone, and androstenedione. In men, there was only a small rise in androstenedione. Levels of sex hormone-binding globulin, estrone, or estradiol did not change in either sex; nor did insulin sensitivity.

Nestler J. *DHEA: Coming of Age.* Ann NY Acad Sci 774:ix-xi, 1995.

Orentreich N, Brind J, Rizer R, Vogelman J. *Age changes and sex differences in serum dehydroepiandrosterone sulfate concentrations throughout adulthood.* J Clin Endocrinol Metab 59:(3): 551-554, 1984. There do not appear to be any changes in levels of DHEAS throughout the months, seasons, or year in men whose levels were tested over a 2 year period.

Ravaglia G, Forti P, Maioli F, Boschi F, Bernardi M, Pratelli L. *The relationship of DHEAS to endocrin-metabolic parameters and functional status in the oldest-old. Results from an Italian study on healthy free-living over-ninety-year olds.* J Clin Endocrinol Metab 81:1173-77, 1996.

Spencer N, Poynter M, Hennebold J, Mu HH, Daynes R. *Does DHEAS restore immune competence in aged animals through its capacity to function as a natural modulator of peroxisome activities?* Ann NY Acad Sci 774:200-216, 1995. The liver of aged rats has decreased numbers of peroxisomes and reduced antioxidant activity. This may lead to increased fatty acid saturation in cell membranes, a decrease in cell membrane fluidity, and a decline in immune function.

Yen SS, Morales AJ, Khorram O. *Replacement of DHEA in aging men and women.* Ann NY Acad Sci 774:128-142, 1995. There was an increase in Insulin-like Growth Factor-I in both men and women after 6 months.

THREE

Your Brain on DHEA

W e all want to feel better. Some people may want to feel better even if it requires the help of a supplement. Is it possible to take a pill on a daily basis and consequently be happier? Starting now?

Scientists now believe that mood, personality, behavior, and thoughts are associated with brain chemicals (neurotransmitters). More than 60 neurotransmitters in our central nervous system have been identified, and undoubtedly more will be discovered in the future. Some of them you may have heard of before, such as serotonin and endorphin, and others may be new to you, such as *norepinephrine*, *DOPA*, *acetylcholine*, and *GABA*.

We now know that nutrients can play a strong role in influencing mood. As an example, the essential amino acid tryptophan, found in protein-rich foods such as eggs, meats, and milk, is used by the body to make serotonin, a neurotransmitter that regulates emotional tone and soundness of sleep.

The importance of tryptophan to the brain does not end with serotonin. After serotonin has been produced, the body can then convert this neurotransmitter to melatonin, a neurohormone that is involved in sleep, immunity, and mood. Melatonin production keeps our daily metabolic rhythms in tune with the day/night cycle and helps keep us deeply asleep during the night. As a consequence of a deep sleep, we feel wide awake and alert the next day, often with a better mood.

Another example of a nutrient that influences the brain is the essential amino acid phenylalanine which is used to make norepinephrine, a neurotransmitter that regulates vigilance (attentiveness), memory consolidation and mood.

As a final example, I should point out that vitamin B6 is a co-factor (necessary catalyst, or helper) for the conversion of tryptophan to serotonin and phenylalanine to norepinephrine. Although plain, ordinary B-complex vitamins are not very glamorous, they are the essential cofactors for the enzymes that drive brain metabolism. Deficiencies of B-complex vitamins are known to cause several serious mental disorders, and daily supplementation has been found to improve mood (Benton, 1995). The question then becomes… Can taking DHEA pills on a daily basis also influence brain chemicals, and consequently our mood, thinking, memory, and even libido?

The adrenal glands make at least 150 different steroid metabolites, including *pregnenolone* and DHEA (see Appendix A for full details of the chemistry). In the past, some of these metabolites were thought to be inactive.

However, we now know that they have a role in influencing behavior and memory. They can act on many receptors in the brain, including GABA (gamma amino butyric acid) and serotonin (Majewska, 1987, 1996). GABA is a brain chemical that inhibits impulses between brain cells (neurons). Drs. Melchior and Ritzmann, from the Department of Psychiatry, Olive View/UCLA Medical Center, in Sylmar, CA, gave 0.5 mg/kg of DHEA to mice and found that it reduced their activity and had a relaxing effect. It is known that DHEA(S) is found in the brain of rats. In fact, some of the cells of the human brain, specifically astrocytes, have the ability to synthesize DHEA (Akwa, 1993). Therefore, DHEA can be considered to be a neurohormone, specifically a neurosteroid (Robel and Baulieu, 1995).

Do you remember what DHEA stands for?

You're thinking, "Okay, I'll buy the mood-influencing part, but are you now going to tell me that DHEA will help enhance my memory to such a degree that I'll be able to remember even the date of my wedding anniversary?"

I can't guarantee DHEA can do this for **you**, but if you have a pet mouse, chances are this hormone can help it find its way around a maze and even help it remember how many holes this morning's piece of Swiss cheese had. Earlier in the chapter I mentioned melatonin, another neurohormone that can influence brain chemicals, mood, sleep, and even dreams. Interestingly, DHEA has been found to have an effect on dreams and memory, too. When 500 mg of DHEA was given to volunteers an hour before bed, there was a significant increase in REM sleep for two hours afterward. REM stands for rapid eye movement, one of the five stages of the sleep cycle, and the stage where dreams occur (Friess, 1994). Dreams are thought to facilitate memory consolidation. In 1988, Dr. James Flood, from the University of California, Los Angeles, School of Medicine, and colleagues, gave injections of DHEA to a group of mice and found the hormone to have significant memory enhancing effects. They conclude, "These experiments open new possibilities for the development of substances that may help in alleviating amnesic disorders in man."

Dr. Flood repeated the study in 1992, this time with pregnenolone, DHEA, and other steroids. Mice were placed in a T-shaped maze and given 5 seconds after a bell sounded to find their way into the correct arm of the T. If they failed to do so within 5 seconds, they were electrically shocked until they succeeded. Once trained in the procedure, the mice were injected with a steroid hormone or a placebo. One week later, they were retested for retention of the learned response.

While many steroids were found to reduce the number of runs required for the mice to relearn the shock-avoidance procedure, pregnenolone and DHEA were exceptional in being active at doses ten to a hundred times lower than any other steroid compound.

The dosage ranges over which different steroids enhanced memory and learning in these mice were unusual. Most steroid hormones were found to enhance learning only within a two- to five-fold dose range. These observations suggest that DHEA and pregnenolone play a special role in the brain.

What about DHEA's influence on the human brain?

Dr. Owen Wolkowitz and Dr. Victor Reus, from the University of California, San Francisco; Dr. Eugene Roberts, from City of Hope, Duarte, CA; and colleagues gave 30 to 90 mg of DHEA per day for four weeks to six depressed subjects, 3 male and 3 female. All six were between 51 and 72 years of age and had low DHEA or DHEAS blood levels. The doses of DHEA used were individually adjusted to bring the levels up to those of young adults.

Therapy with DHEA led to significant increases in serum levels of DHEA and DHEAS. Multiple psychological tests were done which showed that the subjects had improvements in memory and mood. In Chapter 2, I also mentioned the study by Drs. Morales and Yen that showed improvement in well-being when volunteers were given DHEA supplements for 3 months.

Perhaps in the future DHEA and other steroids can have a role in a variety of neurological conditions, such as Huntington's disease (HD), Parkinson's, and Alzheimer's. HD is genetically inherited and occurs in 5 out of 100,000 humans. Symptoms, which consist of dementia (loss of mental powers) and chorea (irregular, jerking movements), often start after age 30. There is no known cure.

Blood levels of DHEAS and cortisol were measured in a group of 11 men with HD and compared to another group of neurologically normal men. DHEA levels were lower in the men with Huntington's disease (Leblhuber, 1995). Whether replacement therapy will be found to be beneficial is not known.

Few studies on DHEA's influence on mood in humans have been published, but there are some in progress, including those by Drs. Wolkowitz and Baulieu.

The experts speak:

Etienne-Emile Baulieu, M.D., Ph.D., Professor, College of France, Paris, and Director of the Institut National de la Sante et de la Recherche Medicale, Department of Hormone Research.

The positive effects of DHEA supplements on well-being, as described by Morales et al, have also been observed in our studies.

Maria Majewska, Ph.D., National Institute on Drug Abuse, Medications Development Division, Rockville, MD.

When a DHEA pill is taken, most of it is first sulfated in the liver before it enters the bloodstream. The majority of the circulating DHEA in the blood is in the sulfated form, which makes it water soluble and difficult to enter the brain. But there is also non-sulfated DHEA circulating in our bloodstream. Since DHEA is lipophilic, meaning it is soluble in fat, it would have little difficulty in crossing the blood-brain barrier. There is no doubt that supplemental DHEA, taken as a pill, can have an influence on our brain.

The full influence of DHEA on neurons and receptors in the human brain is not known, but there is early evidence to suggest that it is GABA antagonistic, that is, it has the opposite effect of benzodiazepines [such as Valium] which are GABA agonists.

DHEA can also be an NMDA agonist [see glossary] which could lead to positive effects such as thinking better and more clearly. Perhaps it can also have an influence on serotonin receptors, hence influence mood. The combination of GABA antagonism, NMDA agonism, and serotonin influences could have a synergistic outcome.

It is also possible that different doses of DHEA will have different influences on mood and alertness. Perhaps starting with low doses, such as 5 or 10 mg, and titrating upwards as needed may be a good idea.

Owen Wolkowitz, M.D., from the Department of Psychiatry at the University of California, San Francisco.

We have found that there is a beneficial response to DHEA supplementation in older patients with low mood who also had low blood DHEA levels. However, our study was small and it was not double blind. We're in the process of doing double blind studies with a larger number of volunteers, ages 50-75. I also think lower, physiological doses are more appropriate than higher doses. More is not necessarily better. Improved mood could be due to the effect of DHEA on GABA receptors and possibly serotonin, too. In addition to better mood, some of our patients have noticed improved libido. Women have noticed their nails to be less brittle and their skin softer.

We are currently studying this steroid in relation to Alzheimer's disease. We don't have any data yet, but I'm optimistic. Perhaps another role for DHEA could be in osteoporosis.

The opinions of clinicians:

Ward Dean, M.D., Pensacola, FL.

The majority of users notice feeling better and having more energy.

Barry Elson, M.D., Northampton, MA.

Positive effects have been more energy and alertness. I would say that about 60% of my patients benefit. I find it also useful in chronic fatigue.

Alan Gaby, M.D., Editor of *Nutrition and Healing* newsletter.

Most users notice enhanced well-being.

Dale Guyer, M.D., Saint Vincent's Hospital, Department of Complementary Medicine, Indianapolis, IN.

Positive effects noted by patients after several weeks include a sense of well-being and better clarity of thought. Some find improvement in sleep patterns, and a few mention that their aches and pains are gone. The latter is a subtle effect.

When we replace DHEA, testosterone levels increase in women, but not much for men. Does it increase libido in women? Absolutely. In men DHEA also increases libido, perhaps not as dramatically.

Davis Lamson, N.D., Kent, WA, has treated several hundred patients with DHEA over the past seven years.

A sense of well-being is common. My patients also tell me that their libido improves and occasionally there is arthritis relief.

Dr. Bob Martin, D.C., a physician in Phoenix, AZ, clinical nutritionist, and nationally syndicated radio talk show host.

I have some very difficult patients who have tried many other therapies without success. I find DHEA can be of great benefit in these patients especially when it comes in improving energy levels, mood, and easing chronic pain.

Christian Renna, D.O., Dallas, TX.

For the past four years I've treated over 100 people with DHEA, mostly for hormone replacement therapy. I am commonly told by my patients that this steroid gives them a sense of well-being. Also common is an increase in libido, more often in women than in men. Occasionally I have found DHEA to be helpful in weight loss.

Gary Ross, M.D., San Francisco, CA.

I use DHEA mostly for people who have fatigue and depression where no other cause can be found. I find it to be absolutely helpful and one of the most useful medicines we have. Some of my patients also notice enhanced libido.

Gerald Sugarman, M.D., Director of Lifetime Wellness in Arroyo Grande, CA, has treated over 100 patients with DHEA.

Common positive effects that my patients tell me are better mood and increased libido.

Jonathan V. Wright, M.D., Tahoma Clinic, Kent, WA. Editor of *Nutrition and Healing* newsletter, and bestselling author of *Healing with Nutrition.*

I started using DHEA back in 1982. The very first patient I treated was a 63 year old office worker. She was unhappily married to an alcoholic, and had been seeing a psychiatrist for the past 10 years for fatigue and a variety of psychiatric problems. I did a complete adrenal panel and found that her DHEA level was very low; to be more accurate, her level was near zero.

I prescribed her DHEA through a compounding pharmacy (it was hard to find any pharmacies that had DHEA at that time). She started taking it and I followed her for a while adjusting her levels, but then she didn't return.

A year went by before she came back to the office. "You know, Dr. Wright," she said with an excited tone, "It's been a productive year. I put my alcoholic husband in a rest home, I stopped going to my psychiatrist, and my boss at work thinks I've taken assertiveness training courses. But hear this... I used to think the rest of the world was oversexed because everywhere you turn around on billboards and TV, there's erotic ads or suggestions. Now that I've been on DHEA, I realize that the rest of the world wasn't oversexed, it's just that the problem was my low libido. I now feel a lot more sensual."

I've treated several hundred patients with this steroid since then. The positive effects of DHEA, such as better mood and better sleep, will be most apparent in older individuals. Women will generally notice greater endurance, strength and stamina, perhaps improved libido. I have not seen any significant influence on libido in men. The effect on younger individuals in their 40s or 50s, unless they have unusually low DHEA levels, will probably not be as noticeable.

Summary

There's early research to indicate that DHEA can improve memory, well-being, and mood, especially in those who have low DHEAS levels. As to libido, one double-blind study of 50 mg for 3 months did not find an improvement, although many patients have reported this to their physicians. Mood elevation will probably be most apparent in those who are already depressed and have low serum DHEAS levels to start with, although even a few people with normal DHEAS levels may notice improved mood or memory. Furthermore,... hm... hm... furthermore,... sorry, but I forgot what I was trying to add.

Martin grinned, satisfied...

So the enhanced well-being and sexual satisfaction I've had since being on this hormone are probably not placebo effects since it seems that some patients have reported the same to their doctors. But what about all the claims I've read in some health magazines that it can prevent cancer and heart disease, lead to weight loss, improve the immune system, and so on... Does the research support these claims?

References:

Akwa Y, Sananes N, Gouezou M. *Astrocytes and neurosteroids: metabolism of pregnenolone and dehydroepiandrosterone. Regulation by cell density.* J Cell Biol 121 (1): 135-43, 1993.

Benton D, Haller J, Fordy J. *Vitamin supplementation for 1 year improves mood.* Neuropsychobiology 1995;32:98-105.

Flood JF, Smith GE, Roberts E. *Dehydroepiandrosterone and its sulfate enhance memory retention in mice.* Brain Research 447:269-278, 1988.

Flood JF, Morley JE, Roberts E. *Memory-enhancing effects in male mice of pregnenolone and steroids metabolically derived from it.* Proc Natl Acad Sci 89:1567-71, 1992.

Friess E, Trachsel L, Guldner U. *DHEA increases REM sleep and changes EEG power spectra in men.* Max Planck Institute of Psychiatry Clinical Institute. Scientific Report: 108-9, 1994.

Leblhuber F, Peichl M, Neubauer C. *Serum dehydroepiandrosterone and cortisol measurements in Huntington's chorea.* J Neurol Sci 132 (1): 76-9, 1995. "These findings may indicate a dysfunction of the hypothalamic-pituitary-adrenal axis and possibly suggest a role of DHEAS as an antiglucocorticoid in HC."

Majewska M. *Actions of steroids on neuron: role in personality, mood, stress, and disease.* Integrative Psychiatry 5:258-273, 1987.

Majewska M. *Neuronal actions of DHEA: Possible roles in brain development, aging, memory, and affect.* Ann NY Acad Sci 774:111-120, 1995. Benzodiazepines and barbiturates are GABAergic agonists and produce memory loss. DHEAS is a GABA antagonist, and should facilitate memory. Those addicted to benzodiazepines are known to suffer from severe memory loss.

Melchior C, Ritzmann R. *DHEA is an anxiolytic in mice on the plus maze.* Pharmacol Biochem Behav 47 (3):437-41, 1994.

Robel P, Baulieu, E. *DHEA is a neuroactive neurosteroid.* Ann NY Acad Sci 774:82-109, 1995.

Wolkowitz OM, Reus VI, Roberts E, Manfredi F, Chan T, Ormiston S, Johnson R, Canick J, Brizendine L, Weingartner J. *Antidepressant and cognition-enhancing effects of DHEA in major depression.* Ann NY Acad Sci 774: 337-339, 1995.

FOUR

TAKE HEART
(BUT DON'T GET A CORONARY)

H eart disease is the leading cause of death in the US. The known ways we can improve our heart health include consuming a high-fiber diet, reducing saturated fat, ensuring a balance of mono and polyunsaturated oils (including the essential fish oils), consuming sufficient dietary *antioxidants* complete with a variety of fresh fruits and vegetables, getting plenty of exercise...you've probably heard all this before. (Philosophical break: Knowledge does not always lead to changes in behavior.)

Is DHEA involved in heart disease?

In 1994, Dr. Laura Mitchell, from the Division of Biostatistics, Washington University School of Medicine, St. Louis, MO, and colleagues, took blood samples of 49 males younger than age 56 who were survivors of a heart attack and compared them to 49 other males of the same age group who had not experienced heart attacks. They found that those with prior heart attacks had significantly lower levels of DHEAS than the controls. They conclude:

These data indicate that serum DHEAS levels are inversely related to premature myocardial infarction in males and that this association is independent of the effects of several known risk factors for premature myocardial infarction.

One of the primary researchers involved in evaluating the association of DHEA and heart disease is Dr. Elizabeth Barrett-Connor, from the Department of Family and Preventive Medicine, University of California, San Diego. She has followed

over 1,000 older men and 942 older women residents of Rancho
Bernardo, CA, some of them for close to 20 years. Her conclusions thus far are that high DHEAS levels are slightly protective of heart disease in men, but not in women. These
conclusions are consistent with results obtained by Herrington
in 1990.

In 1995, Dr. Herrington, from the Section of Cardiology,
Bowman Gray School of Medicine, in Winston-Salem, North
Carolina, published some additional studies correlating DHEAS
blood levels with the level of premature atherosclerosis
(hardening of the arteries) in 206 patients who were under age
50. These patients were given an elective *coronary* angiography
(a special test where a dye is placed in the bloodstream and an
x-ray is taken of the coronary arteries to see how much plaque
has accumulated). They also had their fasting DHEA and
DHEAS levels tested.

Three physicians who did not know the results of the DHEA
levels evaluated the results of the coronary angiographies. The
levels of DHEAS were lower in the men who had coronary artery
disease. Dr. Herrington reports:

*These data lend further support to the clinical and epidemi-
ologic, animal model, and tissue culture studies suggesting that
DHEA may play an important role in the pathogenesis* [cause]
of coronary disease.

However, as Dr. Herrington alludes to in his article, this
information does not give us a clear clue whether low DHEAS
levels cause heart disease or whether heart disease causes low
DHEAS levels. In my opinion, the former is more likely to
be true.

There are at least two possible ways that DHEA could reduce
the rate of heart attacks: As a blood thinner, and by reducing
cholesterol levels.

DHEA as blood thinner

One of the major causes of heart attacks is clots that form in the coronary arteries which reduce or stop blood flow, and thus oxygen delivery, to a major section of the heart muscle. Therefore, medicines that are blood thinners (anti-clotting agents) are often prescribed to patients who have had heart attacks, or even recommended to those with risk factors for coronary artery disease such as smokers, those with high blood lipid levels, and individuals who are already experiencing chest pains. (Aspirin is an example of a blood thinner that many people know about. It has excellent anti-clotting properties, even when adults take the 80 mg dose typically used for children.)

Drs. Jesse, Loesser, and colleagues, from Medical College of Virginia in Richmond, gave 5 healthy young men 300 mg of DHEA three times daily for 14 days and tested their *platelets*. The results were compared to another 5 men who received placebo pills. Four out of the five men on DHEA had platelet aggregation rates prolonged. In other words, it took their blood longer to clot. This anti-platelet activity would be considered beneficial in patients who are prone to heart attacks.

Cholesterol is lowered

We've all heard a zillion times that high cholesterol levels in our bloodstream are not good for us. They can lead to cholesterol sticking to the walls of our arteries and reducing the opening through which our blood can flow– much like how hot water pipes get clogged by rust. The reasons for cholesterol sticking to the walls are many; however, one factor that has not been emphasized adequately by some doctors is oxidation. When cholesterol gets oxidized, it sticks to the arterial walls more easily. Antioxidants, such as vitamins C and E, and especially the hundreds of nutrients found in our fruits and vegetables, can help protect cholesterol from oxidation. Carotenoids and flavonoids are some of the hundreds of plant chemicals found in our produce that have excellent antioxidant abilities. Many of them are also thought to have anti-bacterial, anti-viral, and anti-tumor properties.

Even though cholesterol is found in the foods we eat, dietary sources of this vital steroid are not crucial. The liver makes large amounts of cholesterol, and its output increases when dietary sources are decreased. Many people are surprised to find that cholesterol is the most abundant steroid made in the human body, and it is a major structural component of all *cell membranes*, including the cells found in the brain (neurons and glia).

There are many types of cholesterol-carrying particles in our blood stream, including HDL (known as high-density lipoproteins, the good guys) and LDL (low density lipoproteins, the bad guys). If the LDL level or the LDL/HDL ratio gets too high, it is important that we take steps to lower it. Can DHEA play a role in this lowering?

Dr. Haffa and colleagues, from the University of Wisconsin in Madison, recruited a group of rhesus monkey volunteers. (The monkeys were promised a week's vacation in a tropical forest of their choice at the conclusion of the experiment.) Six of these monkeys were given 60 mg/kg/day of DHEA for 4 weeks (similar to 4000 mg/day for a 150 pound human). The dose was then increased to 75 mg/kg/day for an additional 4 weeks. A control group of 6 monkeys received placebo pills for the full eight weeks. Activity, insulin, and cortisol levels and body weight did not change throughout the study period. At the end of the study, the DHEA-treated monkeys had lower levels of cholesterol than the untreated group. The fraction of the cholesterol lowered was the LDL type, the one that oxidizes most easily and has potentially harmful effects on our circulatory system.

Rabbit owners, take heart!

Rabbits from a strain that genetically has high cholesterol levels underwent heart transplants (Rich, 1993), receiving them from a strain of rabbits with normal hearts. The coronary arteries of the transplanted hearts normally form cholesterol plaques very quickly. One group of rabbits received DHEA supplements after the surgery while the other served as controls. DHEA administration significantly slowed the progression of atherosclerosis (hardening of the arteries).

There have been no formal studies published on the evaluation of coronary arteries in humans after DHEA administration.

The latest human study

At a meeting of the American Heart Association in San Francisco in March of 1996, Dr. Henry Feldman reported a study of 1,709 men aged 40 to 70 who had their DHEAS levels tested. Those with the lowest levels of this steroid were the most likely to have had heart disease, even after controlling for other risk factors such as smoking and diet (*Medical Tribune*, April 4, 1996, page 1). In the same article, Roger Blumenthal, M.D., from Johns Hopkins University in Baltimore, is quoted:

Perhaps DHEA supplements might be used to decrease the risk of male heart disease, just as in females taking postmenopausal estrogen seems to have a benefit. However, that question cannot be answered conclusively until clinical trials are performed to assess the risks and benefits of DHEA therapy.

More opinions from experts:

Elizabeth Barrett-Connor, M.D., Department of Family and Preventive Medicine, University of California, San Diego.

There is yet no evidence DHEA or DHEAS has heart protective effects for women. It may be good for men, but clinical trials are needed.

Michael Bennett, M.D., Department of Pathology, University of Texas Southwestern Medical Center in Dallas.

The epidemiological evidence indicates that males with low DHEA levels have more cardiovascular diseases. Hence, they may benefit with supplementation.

David Herrington, M.D., Division of Cardiology, The Bowman Gray School of Medicine, Winston-Salem, NC.

There is no justification to supplement with DHEA at this time since there is no conclusive evidence that taking DHEA will decrease the rate of heart disease, both in men and women. In my view, public access and use to drugs and food supplements for presumed health benefits should be allowed only when there is conclusive evidence that they are effective.

There is, though, sufficient evidence that DHEA can be beneficial to warrant further investigation. We need the results of large scale clinical trials before making any recommendations.

Robert Jesse, Ph. D., M.D., Director of the Acute Cardiac Care Program, Medical College of Virginia, Richmond.

There are a lot of promising pieces of information that indicate DHEA to have a protective role in the progression of heart disease. It acts as an anti-platelet agent, reduces cholesterol, and may prevent atherosclerosis, although we don't know the full details. It would certainly be reasonable to use DHEA supplements in older individuals to get the levels back to those in youth.

Joseph Mortola, M.D., Department of Reproductive Endocrinology, Beth Israel Hospital and Harvard Medical School, Boston, MA.

We're not sure yet in women, but in men there is strong indication that this steroid can have protective effects; it may even be better than taking vitamin C; it certainly can't hurt. The appropriate dosages, though, have not yet been worked out.

The limited clinical experience we have with humans does not show it to have any significant side effects, at least in the short-term. However, we still need some good studies in order to make more definitive recommendations.

One practical way DHEA could be used is in people who have had heart transplants. Generally their new heart, often from a younger person, starts becoming old fast. Perhaps supple-

menting heart transplant patients with DHEA could allow the hearts to function better longer by reducing the process of atherosclerosis.

DHEA's beneficial influence with heart disease will probably be more apparent in men than in women.

Summary

The data thus far indicate that there is an association between low serum DHEAS levels and heart disease, especially in men. It is possible that supplementation with DHEA can slow the onset of coronary artery disease, but this remains to be fully evaluated. Perhaps supplementation can be beneficial in older individuals, people whose DHEAS levels are very low, and patients who already have heart disease.

DHEA supplementation is only one aspect of a complete healthy heart program and should certainly not be done as compensation for continuing detrimental coronary-artery clogging habits such as chain-smoking or consuming a nutrient-depleted (processed/fast food) diet. The first paragraph of this chapter alluded to some positive dietary recommendations. Here are ten healthy heart tips for everyone, especially those with a tendency for coronary artery disease:

1) Engage in moderate physical activity on a daily, or at least three times a week, basis.

2) Get a deep sleep each night. Occasional melatonin use can be helpful. In addition, melatonin is an antioxidant, although its antioxidant effects may only last overnight.

3) Avoid excessive smoking or alcohol consumption.

4) Maintain normal blood pressure, preferably with diet and exercise, but also with medicines if natural methods are not effective.

5) Minimize chronic stress. Maintain a positive attitude, have warm relationships and try go through life with little anger

or hostility. Our thoughts and moods (brain chemicals) do influence our physical health, including our organs, immune system, and the rest of our nervous system and cells (read *Be Happier Starting Now* for details). There is a direct brain-body and body-brain connection. Our brain releases chemicals and hormones that can influence our physical health, and in turn our body releases chemicals and hormones that can influence our brain. Many researchers and physicians now agree that the brain/body split is over. The field that studies this connection is known as psychoneuroimmunology.

6) Eat plenty of fiber, especially through complex carbohydrates such as grains and legumes.

7) Consume plenty of fresh fruits and vegetables. Variety is key since each one contains a different carotenoid or flavonoid. Maintain a good balance between saturated, monounsaturated, and polyunsaturated/fish oils. Avoid extreme fad diets.

8) Use supplemental vitamins, especially the antioxidants such as C and E. Other antioxidants to consider (there are many of them to choose from) include N-acetyl-cysteine, N-acetyl-carnitine, and coenzyme Q-10.

9) If you're female, consider estrogen replacement after menopause. The ideal dosages, combinations, and forms (estrone, estradiol, estriol, or horse estrogens as provided by Premarin [obtained from horse urine]) are still debatable. Estrogen is also believed to protect against tooth loss by maintaining bone mass in the jaw (*Journal of the American Dental Association*, March, 1996).

10) A blood thinner such as aspirin should also be considered.

Discuss all the above with your physician before making any sudden changes in your habits.

The April 4, 1996, issue of *Medical Tribune* briefly mentioned a study done in Boston that showed 2,000 mg of vitamin C to improve blood flow, and possibly prevent heart attacks, in people with coronary artery disease. Their vessels even dilated. In a randomized, controlled study published in 1996, vitamin E, 400 units a day, substantially reduced the rate of myocardial infarction (heart attack) in those who were proven by angiography to have symptomatic coronary atherosclerosis (plaques). The beneficial effects were apparent within one year of therapy (Stephens).

I predict that DHEA supplementation will likely end up having a role to play in the prevention of heart disease. However, the research is still so early that it is best to first concentrate on the above, more proven strategies. If the above-listed positive habits are already part of your health program, and you want to go beyond, then a discussion with your physician may be appropriate regarding the addition of DHEA to your regimen. It's possible that women who are already on estrogen may need to reduce their dose since DHEA has estrogenic effects.

References:

Barrett-Connor E, Goodman-Gruen, D. *The epidemiology of DHEAS and cardiovascular disease*. Ann NY Acad Sci 774:259-270, 1995.

Haffa AL, MacEwen EG, Kurzman ID, Kemnitz JW. *Hypocholesterolemic effect of exogenous DHEA administration in the rhesus monkey*. In Vivo 8:(6):993-7, 1994.

Herrington D. *DHEA and coronary atherosclerosis*. Ann NY Acad Sci 774:271-280, 1995.

Herrington D, Gordon G, Achuff J. *Plasma DHEA and DHEAS in patients undergoing diagnostic coronary angiography*. J Am Coll Cardiol 16:862-870, 1990.

Jesse R, Loesser K, Eich D, Qian YZ, Hess ML, Nestler JE. *Dehydroepiandrosterone inhibits human platelet aggregation in vitro and in vivo*. Ann NY Acad Med 774:281-290, 1995.

Mitchell LE, Sprecher DL, Borecki IB, Tice T, Laskarzewski P, Rao DC. *Evidence of an association between DHEAS and nonfatal, premature myocardial infarction in males.* Circulation 89:91-93, 1994.

Mohan P. Jacobson M. *Inhibition of macrophage superoxide generation by DHEA.* Am J Med Sci 306(1):10-5, 1993. "The anti-atherosclerotic effect of DHEA may be the result of inhibition of superoxide generation in macrophages."

Rich DM, Nestler JE, Johnson DE, Dworkin GH, Ko D, Wechsler AS, Hess ML. *Inhibition of accelerated coronary atherosclerosis with dehydroepiandrosterone in the heterotopic rabbit model of cardiac transplantation.* Circulation 87 (1):261-9, 1993.

Stephens NG, Parsons A, Schofield P, Kelly F, Cheeseman K. *Randomized controlled trial of vitamin E in patients with coronary disease: Cambridge Heart Antioxidant Study (CHAOS).* The Lancet March 23, 347:781-86, 1996.

FIVE

DHEA AND IMMUNITY

After heart disease, cancer, and stroke, the other leading causes of death in the US are due to infections. As we go on in years, our immune system doesn't work as well. Since DHEA(S) levels decline with aging, and due to promising results in animal studies, it has been suggested that supplementation in older individuals could improve certain functions of the immune system.

There are many types of immune cells traveling in our bloodstream. You have heard of white blood cells. *Lymphocytes* are a type of white blood cell that have multiple functions, including forming antibodies to fight off germs and being constantly on the lookout for any cells in our bodies that could be turning cancerous. When these abnormal cells start growing, our lymphocytes go on a search and destroy mission. Two major types of lymphocytes are T cells and B cells. *Natural killer cells*, *macrophages*, and *monocytes* are other cells that are part of the immune system.

The immune system also produces a number of substances that are involved in keeping us germ-free. Some of the names you have heard of before, such as *antibodies* and *interferon*; others may be new to you, such as *lymphokines*.

In order for a hormone to influence immune cells more effectively, it is important that there be sites on the cell where it can attach. These areas are called *receptors*. Researchers from Kyushu University in Fukuoka, Japan, have found receptors for DHEA on our T cells (Okabe, 1995).

Some studies on DHEA's influence on the immune system of rats look promising. Dr. Rasmussen and colleagues, from Utah State University, wanted to find out if DHEA supplementation would aid rats whose immune system was suppressed by dexamethasone, a powerful steroid that interferes with the proper functioning of B cells, T cells and *immune globulins*. After being given dexamethasone, these immune-suppressed rats were found to be infected with a parasite called cryptosporidium parvum. When the rats received DHEA, most aspects of their immune system normalized and they exhibited significant improvement in fighting the parasitic infection.

Human studies

Nine healthy elderly men with an average age of 64 years took 50 mg nightly of DHEA for 20 weeks (Yen, 1995). DHEA treatment significantly elevated natural killer cells. These are lymphocytes that are involved in searching out and destroying not only viruses, but abnormal cells that are on their way to turning cancerous. Although the number of T lymphocytes was unaffected, T cell function was increased (as measured by an increased proliferative response to phytohemagglutinin, a chemical that normally stimulates T cells). B cell function was also increased.

Vaccines and DHEA

As we age, we make fewer antibodies. Vaccines that are given to the elderly to protect them from influenza, pneumonia, and hepatitis, are sometimes not effective (Miller, 1989).

Drs. Araneo and Dowell, from Paradigm Biosciences, Dr. Woods from University of Utah in Salt Lake City, and colleagues, vaccinated a group of elderly volunteers (age over 65) with the influenza vaccine and compared them to another group similarly vaccinated but who also received 50 mg of DHEAS [sic] for two consecutive days beginning on the day of the vaccination. There was a clear difference: the elderly who got the DHEAS had a significant improvement (fourfold increase) in their ability to develop antibodies to the influenza vaccine. In earlier studies these researchers had found that DHEAS supplementation

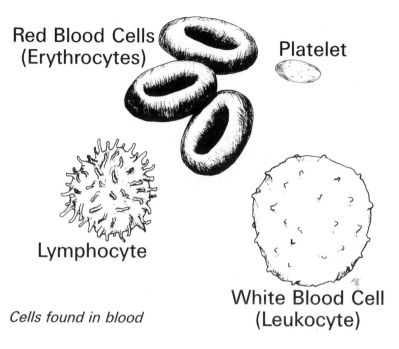

Red Blood Cells (Erythrocytes)

Platelet

Lymphocyte

White Blood Cell (Leukocyte)

Cells found in blood

enhanced the ability of T cells to produce strong antitumor and antiviral chemicals known as interferon and *interleukin-2*.

If further studies support these findings, it may be appropriate to give the elderly a short course of DHEA at the time of vaccination with not only influenza vaccine, but with *pneumococcal* vaccine, tetanus, and others.

AIDS

After an individual is infected with HIV (human immunodeficiency virus), there is usually a period of gradual immune decline eventually reaching a stage of very low immune status– making the body highly susceptible to a number of viruses, bacteria, fungi, and parasites. This low immune state is known as AIDS (acquired immune deficiency syndrome). There are multiple factors that are associated with the progression to AIDS, including nutritional deficiencies and diminished resistance to oxidative stress. (One study has shown that vitamin E may be helpful [Wang, 1994]. Could other antioxidants or nutrients be helpful, too?)

I mentioned earlier that T cells are an important part of the immune system. There are a number of T cells, each with a different name and function. HIV usually infects a type of T cell called helper/inducer (also referred to as CD4). As a consequence, the AIDS patient becomes very susceptible to organisms that a healthy immune system fights off very easily. The term 'opportunistic infections' is given to these bacteria, viruses, fungi, or parasites.

Individuals with normal immune systems will have a CD4 count of over 800 cells per milliliter of blood, whereas HIV infected individuals with opportunistic infections have a count of less than 200.

Dr. Wisniewski and colleagues, from Louisiana State University Medical Center in New Orleans, evaluated the blood levels for cortisol and DHEAS in 98 adults with HIV. There was a significant correlation between DHEAS and CD4 levels, but not between cortisol and CD4 levels. Those who had low DHEAS levels also had low levels of CD4. They conclude:

The data exhibit a positive relationship between the immune status of patients with HIV-related illness and DHEA, leading to the hypothesis that DHEA deficiency may worsen immune status.

We also know that the adrenal cortex of individuals with HIV is commonly infected with the virus. Autopsies performed on patients who died from AIDS have shown that in more than half of the cases, the adrenal glands had been infected with an opportunistic fungus, *mycobacterium*, or *cytomegalovirus* (Rotterdam, 1993). Some even had cancers of the adrenal glands. Over many years of the illness, it would be likely that secretion of DHEA(S) would be lowered.

Does this mean that if DHEA were given to patients with AIDS their symptoms would improve? Or might DHEA supplementation slow the progression of HIV infection to AIDS?

Dr. Dyner and colleagues, at the California Pacific Medical Center in San Francisco, gave between 750 mg and 2,250 mg of DHEA for 16 weeks to 31 HIV infected men with CD4 counts between 250 and 600 cells/ml. The hormone was well-tolerated and no side effects were found. However, there were no improvements in CD4 counts. We do not know whether lower doses of supplemental DHEA may have given different results. We also do not know how DHEA will influence other aspects of the immune system in individuals with AIDS.

DHEA, though, has been found in one small study to correlate with cognitive function (Schifitto, 1996). Six patients (5 men and 1 woman) with HIV, ages ranging from 30 to 51 years, had their DHEAS levels measured. Lower DHEAS levels were associated with more cognitive impairment. The researchers conclude:

Our preliminary data encourage further investigation of the relationship between DHEAS levels and HIV-associated cognitive impairment. DHEAS may represent a useful metabolic marker in combination with neurologic and neuropsychologic examination, in the evaluation of HIV-infected individuals with cognitive complaints.

Natural immune enhancement

There are many ways to improve your immune system. Deep sleep, moderate exercise, travel, relaxation, variety of fresh fruits and vegetables, low stress, positive attitude, multivitamins and minerals (especially C, B, and zinc), and certain antioxidants are a few of the accepted ways. Certain herbs, such as echinacea and goldenseal, also have their believers. Chronic stress is known to impair the immune system, partly since stress increases the adrenal glands' output of cortisol. This adrenal steroid causes significant immune system depression.

Michael Bennett, M.D., from the Department of Pathology, University of Texas Southwestern Medical Center in Dallas, is an expert on DHEA's role in immunity.

DHEA, without a doubt, improves the immune system in aging rodents. We do not have any results of long-term studies in humans, therefore it is anybody's guess how continuous use of this supplement will influence the human immune system when given for a few months or years. In studies on rodents, DHEA counteracts the immune-suppressing effects of glucocorticoids, such as cortisol, and the effects of infectious agents, such as viruses.

Summary

DHEA could, in the future, be found useful as a regular supplement in the elderly in order to boost the immune system. One practical application would be its use in combination with vaccines.

The role of DHEA in the therapy of HIV infection or full blown AIDS remains to be elucidated. A potential help could be in its use to slow or prevent the neurological decline common with this condition.

Perhaps this steroid can be temporarily used during periods of extreme emotional or physical stress in order to counteract the high immune-suppressing actions of cortisol released in response to the stress.

References:

Araneo B, Dowell T, Woods B, Daynes R, Judd M, Evans T. *DHEAS as an effective vaccine adjuvant in elderly humans.* Ann NY Acad Sci 774:232-248, 1995.

Dyner TS, Lang W, Geaga J, Golub A, Stites D, Winger E, Galmarini M, Masterson J, Jacobson MA. *An open-label dose-escalation trial of oral DHEA tolerance and pharmacokinetics in patients with HIV disease.* J Acquir Immune Defic Syndr 6(5):459-65, 1993. There were also no decreases in serum p24 antigen or beta-2 microglobulin levels, but serum neopterin levels decreased transiently by 30%.

Miller R. J Gerontol 44:34-38, 1989.

Okabe T, Haji M, Takayanagi R, Adachi M. *Upregulation of high-affinity DHEA binding activity by DHEA in activated human T lymphocytes.* J Clin Endocrinol Metab 80 (10):2993-6, 1995.

Rasmussen K, Martin E, Healey M. *Effects of DHEA in immunosuppressed rats infected with Cryptosporidium parvum.* J Parasitol 79(3):364-70, 1993.

Rotterdam H, Dembitzer F. *The adrenal gland in AIDS.* Endocr Pathol 4:4-14, 1993.

Schifitto G, Keiburtz K, Palumbo D, Zimmerman C. *DHEAS: a potential metabolic marker of HIV-1-associated cognitive/motor complex.* Neurology 46:A465, 1996.

Spencer NF, Poynter ME, Hennebold JD, MU HH, Daynes RA. *Does DHEAS restore immune competence in aged animals through its capacity to function as a natural modulator of peroxisome activities?* Ann NY Acad Sci 774:200-216, 1995. "We believe that DHEAS facilitates beneficial influences on the immune system through its capacity to control normal peroxisome activities which, in turn, regulate the fatty acid composition of membrane phospholipids and sphingomyelins in lymphocyte and macrophage membranes. The effects of DHEAS on peroxisome function in aging might represent the elusive linchpin needed to provide investigators with a cohesive explanation for the diverse biologic activities of this steroid.

"Immune cells from aged animals and humans often show a decreased ability to synthesize interleukins 2 and 3, whereas the capacity to produce interleukins 4, 5, 6, and 10 is increased."

Wisniewski TL, Hilton CW, Morse EV, Svec F. *The relationship of serum DHEAS and cortisol levels to measures of immune function in human immunodeficiency virus-related illness.* Am J Med Sci 305(2):79-83, 1993.

Wang Y, Watson R. *Potential therapeutics of vitamin E in AIDS and HIV.* Drugs 48(3):327-338, 1994.

Yen SS, Morales AJ, Khorram O. *Replacement of DHEA in aging men and women.* Ann NY Acad Sci 774:128-142, 1995.

SIX

AUTOIMMUNITY AND LUPUS

Our immune system is always on the lookout for any viruses or bacteria that insist on invading our bodies and setting up camp. These germs are quickly told that they are not welcome... and then promptly destroyed.

There are times, though, that our immune system malfunctions. Two different types of mistakes that can be made are: 1) a foreign organism is not recognized as such and allowed to squat and set up camp, and 2) the body's tissues and cells are mistakenly identified as foreign and are mercilessly attacked. This latter mistake is known as autoimmunity (immunity to self). There are many autoimmune conditions including systemic lupus erythematosus, idiopathic thrombocytopenic purpura, multiple sclerosis, pemphigoid and pemphigus, polymyositis, primary biliary cirrhosis, rheumatoid arthritis, scleroderma, Sjorgen's syndrome, and Graves' disease (the most common cause of hyperthyroidism).

Systemic lupus erythematosus (SLE) is four times as common in women as in men. Symptoms include painful and swollen joints, skin rash, and mouth ulcers. A special blood test, called the antinuclear antibody test, is used for diagnosis. SLE is more common than previously thought. A recent study in England showed that up to 200 women out of 100,000 reported symptoms indicative of the illness (Johnson, 1996).

Dr. Suzuki and colleagues, from St. Marianna University School of Medicine in Kangawa, Japan, have found that nearly all of the patients with SLE that they have examined have had low levels of DHEA. In a test tube, they found providing DHEA to the lymphocytes of the patients restored a powerful immune chemical known as interleukin-2. They conclude, "These results indicate that defects of interleukin-2 synthesis of patients with SLE are at least in part due to the low DHEA activity in the serum."

But, practically, do DHEA supplements help patients with SLE?

Dr. van Vollenhoven and colleagues, from the Division of Immunology and Rheumatology at Stanford University Medical Center in California, attempted to learn whether DHEA had clinical benefits in this condition. Ten female patients with mild to moderate SLE were given 200 mg a day of DHEA for 3 to 6 months. After completion of DHEA therapy, most of the symptoms were improved. The women required less cortisone (an immune-suppressing steroid that decreases the symptoms of autoimmune disease). Before DHEA supplementation, three of the ten patients had marked protein loss in their urine which indicates kidney damage. Two of these 3 women showed noticeable improvement on DHEA while the other showed a slight benefit. Except for mild acne-type skin eruptions, the treatment with DHEA was well-tolerated. The researchers propose, "DHEA shows promise as a new therapeutic agent for the treatment of mild to moderate SLE. Further studies are warranted."

Rheumatoid Arthritis

This is a chronic inflammatory disease of unknown origin, with a strong genetic component, that has a tendency to involve joints leading to joint destruction, deformity and loss of function. Rheumatoid arthritis (RA) afflicts about 2% of the population, being more common in older women. In addition to joint involvement, patients also often experience fatigue and depression.

Researchers at the University of Bellvitge, in Barcelona, Spain, evaluated bone mineral density, levels of testosterone, and DHEAS in a group of 99 men with RA and compared them with another group of men of similar age who did not have this condition (Mateo, 1995). There was reduced bone mineral density in men with RA and also reduced levels of testosterone and DHEAS.

Men who had been on corticosteroids also had decreased levels of DHEAS.

Pemphigus and Pemphigoid

These are autoimmune skin diseases that lead to blistering on the skin. Blood levels of DHEA(S) were measured in 21 men and 29 women with these skin problems and compared to 20 patients with psoriasis and 23 with osteoarthritis (de la Torre, 1995). Psoriasis and osteoarthritis are not autoimmune diseases. The average levels of DHEAS were markedly lower in the pemphigoid/pemphigus group. The researchers conclude, "These low levels are consistent with those reported for SLE, RA and polymyalgia rheumatica/giant cell arteritis. DHEAS deficiency is a permanent feature in these autoimmune diseases, and may contribute to their etiology [cause] and/or pathophysiology."

Opinions of...

Ron van Vollenhoven, M.D., Ph.D., a researcher at the Division of Immunology and Rheumatology, Stanford University Medical Center, CA, is one of the world's experts on the role of DHEA with lupus. He told me:

Lupus is one of the conditions where DHEA seems most promising. The reason this condition is more common in women is that it is influenced by hormonal levels, and something about the different hormonal milieu in women makes them more likely to have lupus. It's hard to say whether other autoimmune conditions, such as rheumatoid arthritis, would be helped by DHEA. The studies on lupus, thus far, have been the only well-controlled ones.

DHEA has a lot of potential. I see it as where cortisol was in the 1950's before we learned to modify the molecule and make more powerful analogs of it that could potentially have fewer side effects.

There are two ways DHEA could be used: (1) as a form of therapy, and (2) as hormone replacement to potentially increase life span. The latter has not been well-studied.

The experience of clinicians (remembering that these are anecdotal):

Dale Guyer, M.D., Indianapolis, IN.

I have noticed dramatic effects in patients with autoimmune conditions such as rheumatoid arthritis, lupus, and ulcerative colitis. Almost all of these patients have improved to some degree or another. DHEA is, of course, a part of the overall treatment. I think low doses, such as 10 mg or 15 mg are fine, although I've use as high as 100 mg.

Ron Hoffman, M.D., New York City, NY.

About 20% of my patients notice some positive effect from DHEA. Patients with autoimmune conditions such as lupus and rheumatoid arthritis have been helped. I've also found it helpful in cases of adrenal suppression due to steroids, patients who have fibromyalgia and severe allergies, and also chronic fatigue, although this condition has a variety of causative agents and DHEA is not a quick fix.

There are drawbacks to the use of DHEA. It's expensive, and for the majority of people it doesn't do much.

Jonathan V. Wright, M.D., Kent, WA.

The most common conditions that are helped are almost all the autoimmune conditions such as lupus, Grave's disease, Crohn's disease, ulcerative colitis, and polymyositis. It's not a magic bullet by itself, but it can work well in combination with other therapies.

References:

de la Torre B, Fransson J, Scheynius A. *Blood DHEAS levels in pemphigoid/pemphigus and psoriasis.* Clin Exp Rheumatol 13(3):345-8, 1995.

Johnson, A. The Lancet 347:367-9, 1996.

Mateo L, Nolla JM, Bonnin MR, Navarro, MA, Roig-Escofet D. *Sex hormone status and bone mineral density in men with rheumatoid arthritis.* J Rheumatol 22(8):1455-60, 1995.

Suzuki T, Suzuki N, Engleman EG, Mizushima Y, Sakane T. *Low serum levels of DHEA may cause deficient IL-2 production by lymphocytes in patients with SLE.* Clin Exp Immunol 99(2):251-5, 1995.

van Vollenhoven RF, Engleman EG, McGuire JL. *An open study of DHEA in SLE.* Arthritis Rheum 37 (9):1305-10, 1994.

SEVEN

CANCER CONTROL

In the early part of 1995, the American Cancer Society estimated that 547,000 Americans would die of cancer that year. The most common causes were expected to be due to:

Males

Lung	33%
Prostate	14%
Colon and Rectum	9%
Leukemias and Lymphomas	8%

Females

Lung	24%
Breast	18%
Colon and Rectum	11%
Leukemias and Lymphomas	8%

(*CA– A Cancer Journal for Clinicians* [American Cancer Society], January/February, 1995.)

As we all know, genetics, smoking, and diet play some of the key roles in the initiation and progression of tumors. Smoking is certainly related to lung cancer; diet is believed to influence breast, colon, and prostate cancers; while genetics has the strongest influence on childhood leukemias and lymphomas. Since the focus of this book is on DHEA and adrenal hormones, how are they involved in cancer?

This issue is very complicated and studies thus far have not been consistent. Even after evaluating estrogen replacement therapy for over two decades we still don't have clear answers. One day you'll hear the news media reporting the results of a study published in a prestigious journal that women who take estrogen after menopause will have a higher risk of breast cancer.

A month later, you'll hear the results of another study, again published in a prestigious journal, that estrogen replacement does not increase the risk of breast cancer. By now you've probably pulled out half of your hair and resigned yourself to the possibility that the next study may show estrogen actually protects against breast cancer.

The December, 1995, issue of the *Journal of the American Medical Association* published the results of a long-term study in women (Helzisouer). Blood samples were collected in 1974 from 20,000 women. By 1989, a total of 31 cases of ovarian cancer were identified. Hormone levels of these cancer patients were matched to a group of women who did not have ovarian cancer, known as controls. Compared with the *controls*, the women who had ovarian cancer had higher androgen levels such as androstenedione and DHEA.

A previous study of women who live on the island of Guernsey (a British island in the English Channel) reported that women with ovarian cancer had lower androgen levels than controls (Cusick, 1983), the opposite finding to the study above.

Let's give medicine a break. It's very difficult and expensive to do long-term studies in humans. It's much easier to do the studies in rodents, but extrapolating these results to humans can sometimes give us false leads. Nonetheless, let's briefly review some of these rodent studies.

The majority of the research done on mice and rats has shown that DHEA inhibits the development of experimental tumors of the liver (Simile, 1995), breast (Schwartz, 1979), lung (Schwartz, 1981), colon (Nyce, 1984), skin (Pashko, 1984) lymphatic tissue (Hursting, 1995), and others. When DHEA was administered for 15 weeks to rats who had liver nodules, there was a marked decrease in the number of these nodules (Simile, 1995). When pregnant rats received whole body irradiation during pregnancy and were then implanted with a diethylstilbesterol pellet (DES is cancer causing) for a period of 1 year, a high incidence (96%) of mammary (breast) tumors was observed. Another group of mice who received the same unpleasant treatment, but were supplemented with DHEA, showed only a 35% incidence of mammary tumors. Dr. Inano, a Japanese researcher, concludes, "These findings suggest that DHEA has a potent preventive activity against the promotion/progression phase of radiation-induced mammary tumorigenesis."

Even though a large number of studies in animals have shown DHEA to protect against cancer, I have chosen not to dwell on these studies because I believe results of experiments involving the administration of hormones to humans can be very different from results of similar experiments involving rodents. This is especially true of DHEA since very little of this steroid is found in the bloodstream of rodents. Therefore, no number of cancer studies with DHEA in rodents will convince me one way or the other about DHEA's role in tumor initiation or growth in humans.

The experts speak:

Michael Bennett, M.D., Department of Pathology at the University of Texas, Southwestern Medical Center in Dallas.

DHEA therapy could have preventive effects in humans, as it does in animals, but I doubt that it can be helpful when the cancer is already full steam ahead.

Joseph Mortola, M.D., Department of Reproductive Endocrinology, Beth Israel Hospital and Harvard Medical School, Boston, MA. When asked "Some people have raised concerns that DHEA can induce prostate enlargement or cancer of the prostate in men. Is this possible?"

I'm not worried that low dose DHEA supplementation will induce prostatic enlargement or cancer since it should generally be considered as an anti-androgen in men.

Arthur Schwartz, Ph.D., Fels Institute for Cancer Research and Molecular Biology, Temple University School of Medicine, Philadelphia, PA.

I don't think DHEA itself will be found to be much help in cancer prevention or therapy; however, I am hopeful that analogs of DHEA, such as fluorinated derivatives, could be used to prevent cancer, heart disease, diabetes, and have other benefits without the negative androgenic effects. Androgenic stimulation can lead to insulin resistance, have adverse effects on lipid profiles, and possibly induce prostatic hypertrophy and cancer. We are starting to introduce these fluorinated analogs into human clinical trials in association with the National Cancer Institute.

The clinicians have opinions, too:

Eric Braverman, M.D., Director of Path Medical/Path Foundation, Princeton, NJ.

We have found DHEA, although not a magic bullet or panacea, to be useful in a variety of conditions such as chronic fatigue, burns, Reiter's syndrome, idiopathic thrombocytopenic purpura, menopause, immune deficiencies, memory problems, and even certain forms of cancer. We've given high doses of DHEA, up to 1,000 mg a day, to some terminal cancer cases, such as pancreatic cancer, and noticed that it was of benefit. Other anecdotal cases include shrinkage of lymphomas. We are experimenting using DHEA in combination with chemotherapy or other modalities.

Dale Guyer, M.D., Saint Vincent's Hospital, Department of Complimentary Medicine, Indianapolis, IN.

DHEA has a role in cancer therapy as an addition to chemotherapy. This steroid is one part of the overall treatment, not a cure-all by itself. I've observed that patients with cancer do better when, in addition to conventional chemotherapy, we also add DHEA and use nutritional therapies such as vitamins, antioxidants and melatonin.

Summary

Too little is known about the role of supplemental DHEA in initiating, preventing, or treating cancer in humans. The experience of some clinicians suggests that DHEA, especially when combined with other therapies, can have a beneficial role.

Unfortunately, the longest double-blind, well-controlled, published studies of DHEA administration to humans have only been 6 months. Since cancer cells often take years to grow into obvious tumors, we haven't had enough time to study the role of DHEA supplements in human cancers. The best we can do is make an intelligent prediction based on the available laboratory and animal data, and also based on our present understanding of the physiological role of DHEA and its metabolites. Could DHEA help prevent certain forms of tumors yet stimulate the growth of others? Could the effects be dose-dependent, such as low doses being protective while high doses are harmful?

Summary of the summary

To be brief, whether long-term DHEA administration to humans will help prevent or induce cancer is, at this time, unclear.

References:

Boccuzzi G, Di Monaco M, Brignardello E. *DHEA antiestrogenic action through androgen receptor in MCF-7 human breast cancer cell line.* Anticancer Res 13(6A):2267-72, 1993. "Androgen receptor activation plays a pivotal role in the inhibitory action of DHEA on the E2-induced MCF-7 growth." (See also Lai reference below.)

Cuzick J, Bulstrode J, Stratton I, Thomas B, Bulbrook, R Hayward J. *A prospective study of urinary androgen levels and ovarian cancer.* Int J Cancer 32: 723-726, 1983.

Helzisouer K, Alberg A, Gordon G, Longcope C. *Serum gonadotropins and steroid hormones and the development of ovarian cancer.* JAMA, December 27, 274:1926-30, 1995.

Hursting S, Perkins S, Haines D, Ward J, Phang J. *Chemoprevention of spontaneous tumorigenesis in p53-knockout mice.* Cancer Res 55(18):3949-53, 1995.

Inano H, Ishii-ohba H, Suzuki K. *Chemoprevention by dietary DHEA against promotion/progression phase of radiation-induced mammary tumorigenesis in rats.* J Steroid Biochem Mol Biol 54(1-2):47-53, 1995.

Lai LC. *Metabolism of DHEAS by breast cysts: possible role in the development of breast cancer.* Cancer Detect Prev 19(5):441-5, 1995. Can DHEA stimulate breast cancer cells? Women with palpable breast cysts may have a higher risk of developing breast cancer according to Dr. Lai, from

Freeman Hospital in Newcastle upon Tyne, United Kingdom. He found high concentrations of androgens and estrogens in breast cyst fluid, which may be implicated in breast tumors. He also found that breast cysts were capable of metabolizing DHEA into androstenedione and testosterone. He concludes, "Steroid metabolism by breast cysts may play a role in the development of breast cancer."

Comments: We should keep in mind that just because something goes on in isolated tissues in a test tube does not necessarily mean that the same metabolic events will occur in a live human being. Whether DHEA supplementation will lead to a higher risk of breast tumors is not known. Perhaps low doses will have no effect, or be protective by blocking estrogen receptors, while high doses may be a stimulant. Who knows? (See the Bocuzzi reference above.)

Nyce J, Magee P, Hard G, Schwartz A. *Inhibition of 1,2 dimethylhydrazine-induced colon tumorigenesis in Balb/c mice by dehydroepiandrosterone.* Carcinogenesis 5:57-62, 1984.

Pashko L, Rovito R, Williams J, Sobel E, Schwartz A. *DHEA and 3-beta-methylandrest-5-en-17-one.* Carcinogenesis 5:463-466, 1984.

Schwartz A, Pashko L. *Cancer prevention with DHEA and non-androgenic structural analogs.* J Cell Biochem Suppl 22:210-7, 1995. "There is some evidence to indicate that DHEA produces its antiproliferative and tumor preventive effects by inhibiting glucose-6-phosphate dehydrogenase and the pentose phosphate pathway. This pathway is an important source of NADPH, a critical reductant for many biochemical reactions that generate oxygen free radicals, which may act as second messengers in stimulating hyperplasia."

Schwartz A, Tannen R. *Inhibition of 7,12-dimethyl(a)antracene and urethan-induced lung tumor formation in A/J mice by long-term treatment with DHEA.* Carcinogenesis 2:1335-1338, 1981.

Schwartz A. *Inhibition of spontaneous breast cancer formation in C3H-A mice by long-term treatment with DHEA.* Cancer Res 39:1129-1132, 1979.

Simile M, Pascale R, De Miglio M. *Inhibition by DHEA of growth and progression of persistent liver nodules in experimental rat liver carcinogenesis.* Int J Cancer 62:(2):210-5, 1995. "These data indicate that DHEA inhibits glucose-6-phosphate dehydrogenase activity in rat liver and in persistent nodules in vivo. This is associated with growth restraint of persistent nodules and results in inhibition of their progression to malignancy."

EIGHT

DHEA AND ASTHMA, BURNS, DIABETES, EXERCISE, OSTEOPOROSIS, PREGNANCY AND LABOR, AND... THE BATHROOM SCALE

It is only a matter of time until we discover exactly what role DHEA, melatonin, and other hormones play in influencing not only life span but how they can be used therapeutically in a variety of human conditions. Until then, I would like to share with you in this chapter what we know so far about DHEA's influence on the rest of the human body. Research in the field of hormone therapy is accelerating. In order to keep you informed of the very latest studies, I have started a newsletter called *Melatonin, DHEA, and Longevity Update.* You can find more information about this newsletter in the back of the book.

Asthma

DHEAS values were measured in 72 asthmatic patients with severe bronchospasm (tightening and spasm of the bronchi [lung tubes]) admitted to the Waikato Hospital in New Zealand (Dunn, 1984). Those who had been on oral steroid therapy (glucocorticoids such as prednisone), as a rule, had lower DHEAS levels.

In 1996, Dr. Weinstein and colleagues, from Providence Hospital in Southfield, Michigan, tested DHEA levels in 22 postmenopausal, asthmatic women and compared them with 22 age-matched, postmenopausal, non-asthmatic women. DHEA levels were lower in the asthmatics. Eight of these asthmatic women were given 3 days of oral beta-agonist stimulants (an example is the medicine albuterol which prevents the spasm of bronchi.) All had increased DHEAS levels. The researchers conclude, "These results indicate that postmenopausal asthmatic women have lower serum levels of adrenally derived sex steroids than their nonasthmatic peers and that this anomaly may be ameliorated by adrenergic stimulation."

Whether DHEA supplements will lead to improvement in symptoms in asthmatic patients has not yet been fully evaluated.

Burns

DHEA and its metabolites have so many functions in the body that they can be used therapeutically in a variety of conditions, including burns. When DHEA was injected within 4 hours of a scald burn in animals, there was marked therapeutic benefit (Araneo, 1995). The benefits accumulated when 1 mg/kg/day was continued for 4 days. Examination of the blood vessels around the burned skin showed that DHEA maintained a positive healing process. Dr. Araneo and colleagues, at the University of Utah School of Medicine, Salt Lake City, conclude, "These findings suggest that systemic intervention therapy of burn patients with DHEA or a similar acting steroid hormone may be useful in preventing the progressive tissue destruction by ischemia [loss of blood supply]."

Diabetes

We all need to have some sugar in our blood to keep us energetic. Too little, called hypoglycemia, leads to tiredness and dizziness. Too much, called hyperglycemia, if continued for a long time, leads to a condition called diabetes. The pancreas (see figure in chapter 1), an organ in the abdomen, is chiefly responsible for maintaining normal blood sugar (glucose) levels. When blood sugar levels rise after eating a meal, insulin is released. This helps the glucose to go into our tissues, thus lowering the levels in the blood. Unfortunately, as we get older, our tissues develop a resistance to insulin and the glucose remains in the blood at a higher level.

Drs. Casson, Faquin, and colleagues, from the University of Tennessee in Memphis, wanted to find out the effect of giving supplemental DHEA on insulin resistance. DHEA at 50 mg a day was given for 3 weeks to 11 postmenopausal women. The results showed that blood levels of DHEAS increased up to two times that of premenopausal levels. The levels of triglycerides declined and DHEA enhanced tissue insulin sensitivity. The authors state, "Fifty mg per day of oral DHEA gives supraphysiologic [above normal] androgen levels; 25 mg per day may be more appropriate. There may be a rationale for postmenopausal replacement therapy with this androgen."

A few months later another study was published, this time with 15 subjects, average age 62 years. Fifty mg of DHEA was given to them at 8 am for 3 weeks (Bates, 1995). The results showed a significant improvement in insulin sensitivity. The researchers report, "If DHEA supplementation in aged subjects enhances insulin sensitivity, DHEA replacement may help attenuate [lessen] age-related increases in insulin resistance."

There are no long-term human studies to indicate whether DHEA will be found to be helpful in diabetics. However, rodent studies and preliminary human research indicate that there is a theoretical basis for DHEA's potential benefits.

Michael Bennett, M.D., Department of Pathology, University of Texas Southwestern Medical Center in Dallas.

DHEA can probably have a positive effect in type II (adult onset) diabetes, but little or no effect on type I (juvenile onset).

Exercise

DHEA places an oxidative stress on muscles in rodents. Dr. Goldfarb and colleagues, from the University of North Carolina at Greensboro, tested 64 rats to determine the effects of vitamin E, DHEA, and exercise on antioxidant status in both muscles and plasma. The results of the study showed that exercise, when combined with DHEA use, caused oxidative stress on muscles, but this stress was prevented by adding vitamin E to the diet of the mice (Goldfarb, 1994).

As mentioned throughout this book, results of studies in rodents with DHEA are not always indicative of what would happen in humans. Still, it wouldn't hurt to take 50 to 100 units of vitamin E a day anyway, even if you're not taking DHEA.

Osteoporosis and postmenopausal maladies

Dr. Nawata and colleagues, from Kyushu University in Japan, tested bone mineral density and DHEAS levels in 120 postmenopausal women (51-99 years old) and found a positive correlation. Women with higher DHEAS levels were more likely to have stronger bones. The same researchers, in a previous study, had found that DHEA administration to ovariectomized rats (rats whose ovaries had been removed) significantly increased their bone mineral density. We know that androgens in serum may be converted to estrogens in peripheral organs, especially in bone. Osteoblasts, cells in our skeletal system that are involved in bone formation, were found to take DHEA and convert it into estrogen. Dr. Nawata condludes, "These results demonstrate that the adrenal androgen, DHEA, is converted to estrone (E1) in osteoblasts, and this is important in maintaining bone mineral density after menopause."

What about women who are already on estrogens– can they also supplement with DHEA?

It's difficult to accurately answer this question. Theoretically, since DHEA is partly converted into estrogens in peripheral tissues, estrogen doses may need to be decreased slightly in order to compensate for the DHEA supplementation.

At the 6th annual meeting of the North American Menopause Society (as reported in *American Family Physician*, Feb. 15, 1996, page 939), there was talk of adding testosterone to the estrogen replacement regimen for women. Twelve women received a daily dose of estrogen (1.25 mg), and 13 women received a daily dose of the same estrogen but combined with 2.5 mg of methyl-testosterone for nine weeks. Both treatments improved physical symptoms of menopause such as hot flashes and vaginal dryness, but only the combined regimen significantly relieved psychological symptoms such as nervousness and irritability. The combined therapy also eased insomnia and fatigue.

Comments: Since DHEA can be converted to both estrogens and androgens, could we, proverbially, "kill two birds with one stone?"

Alan Gaby, M.D., author of *Preventing and Reversing Osteoporosis* (Prima, Rocklin, CA).

Although testosterone and DHEA are considered androgens ("male hormones"), they are each produced in substantial amounts by the ovaries. Both of these hormones are considered "bone builders" in that they stimulate the formation of new bone. DHEA levels are frequently low in post-menopausal women.

When androgen deficiency is identified, supplementing with the appropriate hormone(s) will sometimes relieve menopausal hot flashes, fatigue, and depression, and improve libido and immune-system function. The potential to improve bone density is an added benefit of these hormones. (From the September, 1995, issue of *Nutrition and Healing* newsletter, 800-528-0559.)

Pregnancy and labor

Twenty-eight healthy pregnant women had their DHEAS levels checked prior to labor (Liapis, 1993). Significantly higher concentrations of DHEAS were found in women who had good cervical ripening. The researchers propose, "The high DHEAS concentration in maternal plasma may play an important role in pregnancy by producing favorable cervical conditions for delivery or by triggering the labor itself."

Have you heard of prostaglandins? They are hormone-like substances present in many tissues and have countless roles including stimulation of intestinal and uterine smooth muscles.

It is believed that prostaglandins are intimately involved in late pregnancy to induce labor. When Drs. Morimoto and Oku, from Osaka, Japan, placed DHEA in samples of uterine muscles in the laboratory, they found that this steroid influenced the production of prostaglandins.

Based on the above evidence, it would seem that DHEA is closely involved in many aspects of pregnancy, and perhaps, once we learn more about its role, we can take advantage of its effects in inducing labor or ripening the cervix faster.

Sweet dreams

We definitely know melatonin influences sleep and dreams. We briefly discussed this issue in chapter 3. (There's also a chapter in *Melatonin: Nature's Sleeping Pill* titled "Dreams Like You've Never Dreamed.") What about DHEA?

A single dose of DHEA, 500 mg, was given to 10 healthy, young men at bedtime (Friess, 1995). The hormone induced a significant increase in REM sleep. REM stands for rapid eye movement, the stage of sleep associated with dreams. During the dream state, all of our muscles are paralyzed, except for our eye muscles which move to watch the visions in the dream. The rest of our muscles are paralyzed for good reason. We certainly would not want to flail our arms and legs in synchrony with our body movements during our dreams. Otherwise, every night, couples sleeping together would have to wear football-like protective gear and helmets.

Outside of REM sleep enhancement, Dr. Friess, who conducted the study, found no other changes in sleep patterns. He had also checked the levels of testosterone, cortisol, and growth hormone and found the DHEA did not affect these measures.

We've heard of occasional anecdotes by DHEA users that they dream more. Here's a typical story by Marshall Noel, M.D., 48, a physician in Fresno, California.

I started DHEA at 50 mg a day, in the morning, after I learned that some of my colleagues were taking it. My initial blood level was normal for my age group, but low compared to youthful levels. After about a week, I noticed having more energy and a sense of well-being. It's been a month now and I've had no side effects. I'm also dreaming more.

One disadvantage of taking DHEA in the evening is that it can act as a mild stimulant in certain individuals.

DHEA and the bathroom scale

You've tried the grapefruit diet, the high-carbohydrate diet, the low-carbohydrate diet, the high-protein diet, and the low-protein diet, the high-fat diet... and every high and low you can think of. Yet, the weight seems to stay on the high side. Can DHEA come to the rescue?

Don't ask the Zucker rats. When lean Zucker rats were given a diet supplemented with DHEA, they had a significant increase in their caloric intake. When obese Zucker rats were supplemented with the hormone, they consumed less calories and lost weight (Wright, 1993). Go figure.

What happens to fat Zucker rats when DHEA is discontinued? Dr. Porter and colleagues, from Louisiana Medical Center in New Orleans, gave DHEA to them for one week. As expected, their food intake slowed. However, within a day of stopping DHEA, they were back to their gluttonous habits.

What happens to our own DHEA levels when we lose weight? Dr. Jakubowicz, from the Medical College of Virginia/Virginia Commonwealth University in Richmond measured the DHEA levels of men and women who lost weight. He found something curious. DHEA levels rose in the men, while they stayed the same in women. Various other studies have shown that men and women do not necessarily metabolize or use DHEA the same way.

In chapter 2, I mentioned the study by Dr. Yen and colleagues who gave 100 mg of DHEA to 16 men and women for 6 months.

At the end of the study, lean body mass showed an increase in both genders.

The reports in the medical literature evaluating the relationship of DHEA to weight have not been consistent. Back in 1990, at the Medical College of Virginia, Dr. Usiskin and colleagues gave 1,600 mg of DHEA to six obese men for 28 days.

In two out of the six subjects, body fat mass was reduced, but, for the group as a whole, neither body fat, total body weight, body fat mass, nor waist-to-hip ratio changed significantly during the study period. Also, there were no changes in tissue insulin sensitivity or serum lipid levels. The conclusion was that short-term administration of DHEA, in high doses, did not have much of an influence on weight.

A few months after this study was published, another one done at the University of Rochester in New York evaluated the administration of 1,600 mg of DHEA for 4 weeks to eight healthy men (Welle, 1990). The researchers did not find that this steroid had much of an influence on weight loss or energy and protein metabolism. Epidemiological studies also do not support the theory, as had been proposed based on animal studies, that high serum DHEA(S) levels protect against obesity and diabetes (Barrett-Connor, 1996).

What about adding DHEA to diet drugs?

Let's get back to the fat Zucker rats. When they're given DHEA, their caloric intake diminishes and there is an increase in the amounts of serotonin in their *hypothalamus*– a small part of the brain involved in satiety. One popular drug used as a diet pill, fenfluramine, also elevates serotonin levels in the hypothalamus, inducing satiety. Drs. Svec and Porter, from Louisiana State University in New Orleans, treated obese and lean Zucker rats separately with large doses of DHEA and fenfluramine and found their intake of calories to decrease only slightly. However, when they combined both the steroid and the drug, there was a profound effect (Svec, 1995). The lean animals decreased their caloric intake by two-thirds while the obese animals nearly stopped eating. Even a hot fudge sundae with fresh bananas and dark chocolate syrup couldn't get them interested. The researchers conclude, "DHEA and fenfluramine form a synergistic anorectic combination that diminishes profoundly the caloric intake of the Zucker rats, both lean and obese. The effect does not show tolerance over 28 days and can cause significant weight loss in obese animals."

In 1995, the FDA approved the combination of two diet drugs, phenteramine and fenfluramine, for the treatment of obesity. Could DHEA be used in combination with lower dosages of these drugs or even replace one of them?

Michael Bennett, M.D., Department of Pathology at the University of Texas, Southwestern Medical Center in Dallas.

There doesn't seem to be a significant effect on weight loss in humans but many strains of rodents will consume fewer calories when on DHEA, at least for a period of a few weeks.

Davis Lamson, N.D., Kent, WA.

I have not seen much weight loss. I think this promise of DHEA has been hyped.

References:

Araneo B, Ryu S, Barton S, Daynes R. *DHEA reduces progressive dermal ischemia caused by thermal injury.* J Surg Res 59(2):250-62, 1995.

Barrett-Connor E, Ferrara A. *DHEA, DHEAS, obesity, waist-hip ratio, and noninsulin-dependent diabetes in postmenopausal women: the Rancho Bernardo Study.* J Clin Endocrinol Metab 81(1):59-64, 1996.

Bates CW, Egerman RS, Umstot ES, Buster JE, Casson PR. *DHEA attenuates study-induced declines in insulin sensitivity in postmenopausal women.* Ann NY Acad Sci. 291-293, 1995.

Casson P, Faquin L, Stentz F, Straughn A, Andersen R, Abraham G, Buster J. *Replacement of DHEA enhances T-lymphocyte insulin binding in postmenopausal women.* Fertil Steril 63(5):1027-31, 1995.

Dunn PJ, Mahood CB, Speed JF, Jury DR. *DHEAS concentrations in asthmatic patients: pilot study.* N Z Med J 97(768):805-8, 1984.

Friess E, Trachsel L, Guldner J, Schier T. *DHEA administration increases rapid eye movement sleep and EEG power in the sigma frequency range.* Am J Physiol 268: E107-13, 1995.

Goldfarb A, McIntosh M, Boyer B, Fatouros J. *Vitamin E effects on indexes of lipid peroxidation in muscle from DHEA-treated and exercised rats.* J Appl Physiol 76(4):1630-5, 1994.

Jakubowicz D, Beer N, Beer R, Nestler J. *Disparate effects of weight reduction by diet on serum DHEA in obese men and women.* J Clin Endocrinol Metab 80(11):3373-6, 1993.

Liapis A, Hassiakos, D, Sarantakou A, Dinas G, Zourlas PA. *The role of steroid hormones in cervical ripening.* Clin Exp Obstet Gynecol 20(3):163-6, 1993.

Morimoto K, Oku M. *Effect of progesterone, cortisol and dehydro-epiandrosterone-sulfate on prostaglandin production by cultured human myometrial cells.* Nippon Sanka Fujinka Gakkai Zasshi 47:391-7, 1995.

Nawata H, Tanaka S, Takayanagi R. *Aromatase in bone cell: association with osteoporosis in postmenopausal women.* J Steroid Biochem Mol Biol 53(1-6):165-74, 1995.

Porter J, Abadie J, Wright B, Browne B, Svec. *The effect of discontinuing DHEA supplementation on Zucker rat food intake and hypothalamic neurotransmitters.* Int J Obes Relat Metab Disord 19(7):480-8, 1995.

Svec F, Porter JR. *Synergistic anorectic effect of DHEA and fenfluramine on Zucker rat food intake and selection: the obesity research program.* Ann NY Acad Sci 774:332-334, 1995.

Usiskin KS, Butterworth S, Clore JN, Arad Y, Ginsberg HN, Blackard WG, Nestler JE. *Lack of effect of DHEA in obese men.* Int J Obes 14(5):457-63, 1990.

Weinstein RE, Lobocki CA, Gravett S, Hum H, Negrich R, Herbst J, Greenberg D, Pieper DR. *Decreased adrenal sex steroid levels in the absence of glucocorticoid suppression in postmenopausal asthmatic women.* J Allergy Clin Immunol 97:1-8, 1996.

Welle S, Jozefowicz R, Statt M. *Failure of DHEA to influence energy and protein metabolism in humans.* J Clin Endocrinol Metab 71(5):1259-64, 1990.

Wright B, Browne E, Svec F, Porter J. *Divergent effect of dehydroepiandros-terone on energy intakes of Zucker rats.* Physiol Behav 53(1): 39-43, 1993.

NINE

WHEN AND HOW MUCH
DOSING MADE EASY

A fter interviewing more than 40 researchers and clinicians familiar with DHEA, I have realized that there is a wide range of opinions concerning testing and dosing. This is because the studies on DHEA in humans are still in their infancy; consequently, the practice of DHEA supplementation is still an art rather than a science. (The practice of medicine is also an art. For instance, if a patient goes to a few different doctors complaining of a particular symptom, there's no guarantee that the diagnosis, lab tests ordered, and methods of therapy will be consistent among all the physicians.)

The following are some general approaches the doctors I interviewed use to evaluate a patient before starting therapy with DHEA.

- A few physicians will not do any testing before initiating DHEA because they claim the blood tests are expensive and inconvenient, and the results inconsistent. These doctors assume that almost all older individuals are low in DHEA(S) anyway, and will prescribe 5, 10, 25, or 50 mg to see if there are benefits. If so, they will continue the therapy. If side effects occur, they will lower the dose.

- The majority of clinicians will check DHEAS levels on almost every patient after a certain age, such as 40 or 50, and then recommend DHEA if levels are low. Some are very conservative in their dosages and will start with 5 or 10 mg initially and titrate up if these doses, after a month or so, do not elevate blood DHEA(S) levels back to youthful levels, or do not provide any noticeable benefits. It seems that experienced physicians are first opting for this conservative low dose approach before moving on to higher doses.

- A rare opinion is that 25 or 50 mg of DHEA will not lead to anti-aging outcomes and perhaps higher dosages, such as 200 mg or more, are appropriate. At least one scientist believes that the DHEA molecule has to be altered, such as being fluorinated, to have a significant influence on longevity.

- And there are also the researchers who think DHEA will do nothing for you, and you might just as well take a sugar pill– it's cheaper (and you also don't need a doctor's visit or blood studies).

As you have already gathered having read thus far into this book, Medicine does not always speak with one voice. Rational, intelligent physicians, looking at the same data, may come to different conclusions. Even after studying the simple vitamins and nutrients such as C, E, and beta carotene for 2 or 3 decades, there is still no consensus among physicians how they influence health and longevity and if so, what dosages are best. It will take us many more decades to sort everything out.

In the meantime, I have chosen in this book to present to you, the intelligent reader, all the options, and let you, in consultation with your personal physician, decide whether DHEA is appropriate for your unique circumstance, and if so, how much.

There are at least two types of individuals and physicians– conservatives who want to patiently wait until all the studies are in before starting a course of action, and adventurists who will take a particular supplement based on an educated guess on its purported benefits from the available, limited studies. These adventurists claim they don't have the patience, or life expectancy, to wait a few decades for the definitive results. Where do you fit in?

Here are some answers to questions I was asked while writing this book.

What forms and dosages does DHEA come in?

Capsules are the most common form. Compounding pharmacies can make them in any dosage that a doctor recommends, from 5 mg to 200 mg. They can also make DHEA creams, ointments, and even lozenges.

If you buy DHEA without a prescription, you can generally find it in 10, 25, and 50 mg capsules.

When a DHEA pill is swallowed, it is first absorbed from the stomach and intestines, then goes through the liver before making its way to the rest of the body. The liver is the chemical factory of the body and it makes good sense for it to have "first crack" at the blood supply from the digestive system. Physicians call this the "first-pass effect."

One of the liver's functions is to metabolize sterols and steroids. Cholesterol is a common dietary sterol and the liver bundles it into lipoproteins (fatty globules) for distribution to body tissues. If there's not enough cholesterol in the foods we eat, the liver makes more of it to make up the difference. The liver also metabolizes DHEA. Because of this, DHEA pills that you swallow will first be metabolized by the liver and the amount that reaches the general circulation will likely be less than the ingested dose. The factors that influence absorption from the intestines and metabolism by the liver vary significantly with age and health condition. Testing (before and after DHEAS levels) may be the only way to know for sure how much is eventually reaching the bloodstream.

One way that pharmacists minimize liver metabolism of steroids is to use "micronized" preparations. Micronization is a process that creates tiny particles that can be absorbed from the intestines into the lymphatic system and partially bypass the liver. Although micronized DHEA is now available, I have seen only limited data supporting its proposed enhanced bioavailability.

John Buster, M.D., Director, Division of Reproductive Endocrinology and Infertility, Department of Obstetrics and Gynecology, Baylor College of Medicine, Houston, TX, has been studying, along with Peter Casson, M.D., the bioavailability of DHEA.

Our studies indicate that micronized DHEA gets absorbed more easily from the intestinal system by being absorbed through the lymphatic system, partially bypassing the liver. This form of DHEA also does not seem to be converted to testosterone as much, thus possibly reducing negative androgenic effects on the prostate gland or lipids (Casson and Buster, 1995).

Another potential route to minimizing liver metabolism of DHEA is by sublingual administration. Sublingual refers to under-the-tongue use which allows a significant amount of DHEA to be absorbed into the tiny capillaries of the mouth whose blood supply passes into the general circulation before going to the liver. Sublingual preparations of many vitamins, drugs, and herbal extracts are common. Even melatonin can be taken sublingually. However, I have not seen any research to indicate whether the sublingual approach to DHEA supplementation is preferable to the oral route. Lozenges are a lot more expensive and unless you have trouble swallowing or have problems with absorption, for now you may do just as well with the capsules.

Ron von Vollenhoven, M.D., Ph.D., Division of Immunology and Rheumatology, Stanford University Medical Center, CA.

It's been difficult to predict serum levels of DHEAS based on dosages from oral administration since the absorption rates are often variable.

What's the best dosage to start with?

There is a wide range of opinions on the ideal starting dosage. I am generally conservative in my approach and prefer most medicines to be started at a low dose. For instance, my feeling about melatonin is that 0.3 mg is a safe dose for the first night. This dose is low– most pills in the vitamin stores are 3 mg. If 0.3 mg is not effective, then it can be increased the following night.

As to DHEA, most of the pills on the market come in 25 and 50 mg. I feel that 5 or 10 mg is a good starting dose. If you can only find the higher dosages, you could open the capsules and take a small portion, saving the rest for following days. Of course, much depends on your initial DHEAS levels, along with your unique rate of absorption and metabolism, and, of course, the advice of your health care provider.

I recommend that you are supervised by a physician familiar with DHEA. If you would like more information on how to find a physician in your area knowledgeable about this steroid, see the back of the book.

What time of day should I take my DHEA?

The adrenal gland makes lots of DHEA in the early (pre-dawn) morning, and production drops dramatically throughout the day. Most doctors recommend taking DHEA in the morning to act in concert with this natural circadian (daily) pattern. Although I am inclined to agree with this, I could not find any data to support morning dosing as being better than other times.

John Buster, M.D., Director, Division of Reproductive Endocrinology and Infertility, Department of Obstetrics and Gynecology, Baylor College of Medicine, Houston, TX.

I'm not aware of any data to indicate what time of day is ideal for dosing.

Christopher Longcope, Ph.D., Department of Obstetrics and Gynecology, University of Massachusetts Medical School, Worcester.

DHEAS levels are generally constant throughout the day, so it really doesn't matter what time of day you supplement with DHEA. Anytime of day would be fine. Moreover, there's no differ-

ence whether you take DHEA or DHEAS pills since the body can interconvert.

When we ingest a pill of DHEA, it gets absorbed from the intestinal tract through the portal vein and on to the liver where it is mostly sulfated into DHEAS. DHEAS will then enter our bloodstream. Only about 10% of the DHEA will circulate in our bloodstream without being sulfated.*

How quickly is DHEA absorbed?

When a group of postmenopausal women were given 1,600 mg of this steroid, DHEA and DHEAS blood levels rose within 60 minutes (Mortola, 1990). There was a rapid rise in androgen levels but a much slower rise in estrogens.

At what age should I get my DHEAS levels tested?

Most physicians who incorporate DHEA replacement therapy in their practice will test people starting in their 40s. If the levels are found to be low, DHEA is started and the levels monitored every month or two until the desired plateau is reached. From then on, DHEA levels are monitored every few months. Some physicians will also order a regular blood test to check levels of other blood chemistries. Just to be completely safe, a few physicians may even do mammograms and pap tests in women and check a prostate cancer blood test (PSA) in men.

A blood test is the standard and routine way to check levels, however, at least one clinical director of a laboratory, Elias Ilyia, Ph.D., from Diagnostechs Labs in Seattle WA, says he has examined tens of thousands of blood and salivary levels and feels saliva tests are simpler and just as accurate. I could not find any published data to determine which method was preferable.

John Buster, M.D., Director, Division of Reproductive Endocrinology and Infertility, Department of Obstetrics and Gynecology, Baylor College of Medicine, Houston, TX.

I am not aware of any data comparing saliva tests versus blood tests. There is a lot we don't know about this steroid. Our knowledge of DHEA is where estrogen was about two or three decades ago.

Another option is a 24 hour urine test to check levels of DHEA and its metabolites such as androsterone and etiocholanolone. According to Dr. Jonathan Wright, one lab, Meridian Valley in Kent, WA, charges about 70 dollars for this urine test. The cost of blood tests varies between different labs, ranging between 40 and 100 dollars.

Over the last ten years serum DHEA and DHEAS testing services have evolved from obscure research tools to readily available clinical tests. Although a lot of doctors have never ordered DHEA(S) levels, more likely than not the laboratory they use for standard blood tests also does testing for this steroid. As testing becomes more common the price will likely decrease.

How are DHEA levels measured?

When a doctor orders a blood test for you, the results will often come back in micrograms per 100 ml, or in micrograms per ml. The laboratory will print on its lab result sheet what the normal ranges are for different age groups. These may vary between different labs. Usual ranges are anywhere from 40 mcg/100 ml which is very low and found in very old people to 450 mcg/100 ml found in certain young people at their prime. Some labs will also provide the results in nanograms per ml. A nanogram is one thousandth of a microgram.

1 mg = 1,000 micrograms (mcg) = 1,000,000 nanograms (ng)
= 1,000,000,000 picograms (pg).

The opinions of experienced clinicians:

Edmund Chein, M.D., Palm Springs, CA.

I always do a blood test before starting DHEA and during the course of replacement to get the levels back up to what they are in our 20s. I use whatever dose it takes to get the levels back to those of youth, which could be as low as 2 mg or as high as a few hundred mg.

Barry Elson, M.D., Northampton, MA.

I've treated about 60 people over the past 3 years. I always do a blood test before starting anyone on it. I use DHEA mostly for patients who are tired and have low energy. My dose is 5-15 mg for women and I gradually increase it as needed.

Alan Gaby, M.D.

I was prescribing 25-50 mg of DHEA but now I've lowered my dosage to 5 to 15 mg in women, and 25 to 30 mg in men. It's possible that higher dosages may be less beneficial than lower dosages, except when treating autoimmune conditions. I've had success with one patient with rheumatoid arthritis whom I switched from prednisone to DHEA. My caution to users is not to take too much of this steroid.

Allen Green, M.D., Medical Director, Institute for Holistic Treatment and Research, Newport Beach, CA.

I use it for hormone replacement therapy and a variety of conditions, including chronic fatigue syndrome, fibromyalgia, HIV and immune enhancement. Since I also use other holistic modalities in addition to the DHEA therapy, it's hard to ascribe the improvement in my patients exclusively to DHEA.

I definitely check DHEA levels initially, and for those who are on hormone replacement therapy for anti-aging purposes. Once the blood DHEAS level become stable, I test it once a year to keep it in the upper normal range of youth.

Douglas Hunt, M.D., Burbank, CA.

I start my patients on 5 mg and work up from there by increasing the dose 5 mg every week or so until there is some noticeable improvement. Some patients report an effect on as low a dose as 2 mg, while others have been on 250 mg without feeling anything.

I've treated more than 200 patients with DHEA over the past 3 years. More and more I'm realizing that lower dosages are more appropriate. I've learned to respect this drug for its power and its strength. It can be overwhelming in some people.

Women can overdose too fast on this steroid and get unpleasant reactions such as fatigue, anger, depression and a variety of emotional symptoms. However, when the right dose is found, DHEA can be an energizer and mood elevator. I use it for assertiveness. On right doses patients report they have more energy and confidence. It's possible careers can improve. I even have patients tell me they have more libido. They volunteer this information without my asking.

I use DHEA in those with chronic fatigue syndrome, often with a combination of B vitamins. For those who complain of low energy late in the day, I recommend the DHEA in the afternoon since it can have a stimulating effect.

I haven't seen any acne or hair growth because I use low doses. In rare cases blood pressure has been elevated. Follow up blood tests have not shown any hormone, lipid, or glucose changes.

Davis Lamson, N.D., Kent, WA.

Testing DHEA(S) levels before starting this steroid is a must. I strive for normalizing the levels of this hormone to those of youth. Using it in combination with estrogen replacement therapy is appropriate.

Lord Lee-Benner, M.D., Newport Beach, CA, author of *Turning Back the Aging Clock* (World Health Foundation, 1990).

I have treated at least 100 patients with DHEA. I initially check blood levels once a month. However, I find them not reliable since I can't seem to get consistent results from the laboratories who are presently doing the assays.

Some individuals will have decreased libido and patients with chronic fatigue syndrome may initially feel better, then after a while the benefits are often gone. Only a small percentage notice improved libido.

I generally try doses such as 10 mg or 25 mg, given twice a day. It's rare that a patient tells me that they benefit from taking it.

When asked "Then why do you keep using it?"

I think it has a role in older people, especially when used in combination with growth hormone. I'm not using it as much on my patients now as I used to.

Christian Renna, D.O., Dallas, TX.

I prefer to use low doses such as 10 mg in women and slightly higher in men. I always do blood tests. DHEA can be combined with estrogen and also testosterone and progesterone. It's important to evaluate levels of all hormones in older individuals and replace the ones that are low instead of just focusing on one.

Gary Ross, M.D., San Francisco, CA.

I start my patients on lower doses such as 5 mg for women and 15 mg for men, with a maximum dose of 30-50 mg. I've used as low a dose as 2 mg. Blood tests are mandatory.

Murray Susser, M.D., Santa Monica, CA.

I use it as hormone replacement therapy in doses of 5 to 25 mg. Many of my patients notice more energy and vitality with better libido. The improved libido occurs especially in women who have low testosterone levels. On the down side, some patients experience tiredness, depression or anger with high doses. There have also been rare cases of fluid retention. I check blood levels every three months.

Karlis Ullis, M.D., Santa Monica, CA.

I'm conservative in my approach with DHEA. Therapy needs to be individualized. Over the past two years I've treated 50 patients with it. For people interested in anti-aging medicine, I routinely do a blood panel of not only DHEA(S), but also total estrogens, estradiol, estrone, and in men, free testosterone. I also check levels of IGF-I (insulin-like growth factor).

If the levels of DHEA are low, I replace it, generally starting with 25 mg, and then titrating up or down. In about 2 months, I will repeat the blood tests to see where the levels of the hormones are.

Some men on DHEA notice decreased libido, increased fat, and decreased muscle fat, perhaps due to the DHEA blocking androgenic receptors. This is why we need to individualize therapy since we don't know, when we give DHEA, which way it will be metabolized in an individual person: whether it will go into an androgenic pathway or estrogenic pathway (Ebeling, 1994).

Many women notice a positive response, such as a boost in energy, drive and well-being, probably correlating with increased androgenic activity. I have not found them to have any lipid changes or insulin resistance. In some of the men I have placed on DHEA, their estrogen levels went up.

Jonathan V. Wright, M.D., Tahoma Clinic, Kent, WA.

DHEA metabolizes into testosterone and many other metabolites. When following women, we test urine androgenic steroids, sometimes doing a full sex steroid profile. We often find elevated testosterone levels in women following DHEA administration. Other female patients will take large DHEA doses, yet their testosterone levels don't budge. In these women, we give them additional testosterone. Every patient is unique, therefore, it's hard to give any specific recommendations.

Before finalizing the appropriate therapeutic dose of DHEA, it is mandatory to check DHEA levels and its downstream metabolites such as androsterone and etiocholanolone. I find 24 hour urine testing to be appropriate for these purposes. Sometimes a dosage of DHEA that will produce a normal range of serum DHEA and normal urinary DHEA will also produce urinary levels of androsterone and etiocholanolone from 3 to 6 times normal levels. This is not physiologic and thus potentially unsafe. The dose of DHEA must be cut back and adjusted until all of these DHEA metabolites are within physiological range.

To do otherwise is incomplete. Current technology allows us to test these levels, and they should be done.

Summary

If you're planning hormone replacement therapy with DHEA:

- Find an experienced health care practitioner to supervise you. If your current practitioner is not knowledgeable about DHEA, give him or her a copy of this book.

- Have your DHEAS levels measured.

- Start on a low dose of 5 or 10 mg. This dose can be increased if subsequent testing shows DHEAS levels have not been elevated sufficiently.

- Feel free to write to me at the publisher's address and let me know about your experience.

References:

Casson PR, Buster JE. *DHEA administration to humans: panacea or palaver?* Seminars in Reproductive Endocrinology 13(4): 247-254, 1995.

Ebeling P, Kolvisto V. *Physiological importance of DHEA.* The Lancet 343:1479-1481, 1994.

TEN

CAUTIONS AND SIDE EFFECTS

I interviewed a large number of researchers and clinicians who are very familiar with DHEA. Their combined experience with thousands of patients does not indicate that DHEA has any serious or toxic effects in reasonable doses. Nonetheless, it is still best that we proceed cautiously until more long-term studies are available.

Side effects noted with high dose DHEA use include:

- acne, generally mild
- hair growth in women (in unwanted places)
- deepening of voice
- irritability or mood changes
- overstimulation or insomnia
- fatigue or low energy

Please note that these side effects are infrequent on doses less than 15 mg, and most users note positive effects. Furthermore, many users do not notice any effect one way or the other. The above side effects quickly disappear upon stopping or reducing the dose of the steroid.

Theoretical risks with long-term DHEA supplementation include an influence on hormone-sensitive cancers such as breast, uterus, ovaries and prostate.

Other theoretical influences with supplementation for many years include effects on blood glucose levels, lipids, and other hormones. The longest well-controlled, double-blind studies to date have only been 6 months. Dr. Baulieu, in Paris, France, is at this time conducting long-term studies on a large number of human volunteers. His results should be published in the next few years.

Acne

Did you ever in your teens wake up in the morning when your very first move was to put your face an inch and a half away from the mirror and microscopically analyze every pore for any new pimples that had blossomed overnight? If you never did, you may start if you regularly take high doses of DHEA.

Stimulation of sebaceous glands by androgens is an important cause for the development of acne. Dr. Walton and colleagues, from Princess Royal Hospital in Hull, England, examined hormone levels in 36 women ages 14 to 34. The hormones checked were testosterone, sex hormone binding globulin, DHEAS, and dihydrotestosterone. They found the levels of DHEA and DHEAS to be elevated in women who had acne.

In another study, when 34 women with adult onset acne were compared to a control group, the ones with the skin condition were found to have an excess of androgens, including DHEA, testosterone, and dihydrotestosterone (Aizawa, 1993). Using a test that determines the source of the excess androgens, the researchers determined that the androgens were coming from the adrenal glands, and not necessarily from the ovaries.

Patients with systemic lupus erythematosus who were given 200 mg a day of DHEA for 3 months were noted to have mild acne rash (van Vollenhoven, 1994).

Low doses of DHEA, such as 5 or 10 mg, will be less likely to induce acne than higher doses such as 25 or 50 mg. Acne with DHEA supplements seems to be more common in women than in men.

Pregnancy

Although we don't know what would happen if pregnant women are given DHEA, we do have an indication that this hormone plays a role in ripening of the cervix, as we discussed in chapter 8.

At this time it would be best not to use this hormone during pregnancy or breast feeding unless you are a part of a well-controlled clinical study.

I heard that rats had liver damage or tumors when given DHEA. Is this true?

A concern that has been raised is that DHEA supplementation can cause liver damage in rats. Thirty-two rats were treated with 100 mg/kg/day of DHEA for 5 weeks. This would be equivalent to giving a 70 kg human 7000 mg. At the end of the study, the rats had their livers checked. There was significant stress on their livers. When another group of rats were given the same treatment but were also supplemented with vitamin E, the stress on the liver appeared to be much less (McIntosh, 1993). Other studies on rats have also indicated liver damage, tumors, or stress with high dose DHEA use (Rao, 1992).

In one species of fish, the rainbow trout, DHEA at a dose of 12mg/kg/day for 7 months also induced liver tumors (Orner, 1995). This dose is equivalent by weight ratio to 840 mg a day for a 70 kg human.

As with any medicine, we have to be very careful in extrapolating from rodent studies to humans since there may be contradictory results from one species to another. As emphasized throughout this book, rodents have little circulating DHEA in their system and therefore any dose given to them would be a pharmacological (unnaturally high) dose.

But to find out for sure, I went straight to the source and asked Dr. Rao, the researcher who had found the liver damage and tumors with DHEA use in rats, and asked him whether he was concerned with potential liver problems in humans with the use of this steroid.

M. S. Rao, M.D., Department of Pathology, Northwestern University Medical School, Chicago, IL.

The risk of DHEA causing liver cancer in humans is nil since none of the peroxisome proliferators cause a substantial increase in the number of peroxisomes in man. It is very species-specific. Even hamsters and guinea pigs do not respond the same way as do mice and rats. Therefore, I am not concerned that DHEA will cause liver damage or tumors in humans.

My guess is that some of you may be quite relieved by this news and will be heading straight to the local bar for a 6-pack cheer.

Do men and women respond differently to DHEA?

In an article published in *The Lancet* in 1994, Drs. Ebeling and Kolvisto, from Helsinki University Hospital in Finland, propose that DHEA can be metabolized into either estrogens or androgens depending on age and sex.

A woman before menopause has high estrogen levels and low androgen levels. DHEA supplementation can decrease the effects of estrogen by binding competitively to estrogen receptors. The potential negative androgenic effects of DHEA (on heart disease) are counterbalanced by the high estrogen levels present already in these women. (Estrogen is protective of the cardiovascular system.)

A woman after menopause has low estrogen levels and low androgen levels. DHEA supplements can bind to vacant estrogen receptors and have an estrogenic effect. The enhanced androgenic effects of DHEA are now not counterbalanced and could theoretically lead to negative effects on lipids and heart disease.

Men have low levels of estrogens and high levels of androgens. DHEA can bind to estrogen receptors and have estrogen-like effects. Perhaps this could be protective of heart disease.

These theories have yet to be proven in actual, long-term human studies. There may also be individual variability within each sex. Also, DHEA could have predominant estrogenic or androgenic effects depending on what dosage is used.

As you can see, it's a little more complicated than we think. This gives further support to the idea of monitoring various sex hormone levels in individuals who are on this steroid.

More opinions:

Christopher Longcope, Ph.D., University of Massachusetts Medical School, Worcester.

If you're going to take it, stay on a low dose until we learn more. High doses given to rats can cause liver damage. Stop if you notice any problems. We don't know the full side effects in the long term, especially whether elevated testosterone levels will lead to prostate enlargement or cancer.

Owen Wolkowitz, M.D., Department of Psychiatry at the University of California, San Francisco.

The only side effects we have noticed are mild headaches, low energy, and, rarely, constipation or diarrhea.

Ron von Vollenhoven, M.D., Ph.D., Division of Immunology and Rheumatology, Stanford University Medical Center, CA.

In our experience, having treated a large number of women with 50 mg to 200 mg of DHEA for close to 3 years, there have been no major side effects. Mild ones have been acne in women (we have had few men in our studies), mild hair growth, and rare cases of menstrual irregularities and mood changes. The blood tests in the patients we have followed on DHEA have been okay, without any apparent changes in liver enzymes.

The clinicians speak:

Eric Braverman, M.D., Princeton, NJ.

Blood levels are necessary for the initial evaluation and follow-up maintenance. I recommend men to have their prostatic surface antigens (PSA) tested since we've noticed that they can become elevated, especially in older men. (PSAs are a marker for prostate enlargement or tumor.) Women should have regular pap tests and mammograms.

Side effects we've seen on higher doses are acne and facial hair in women, sometimes on the chin [not a popular side effect]. *I don't advise people with liver disease to take DHEA since the liver is where this steroid is sulfated after we ingest it.*

Positive effects that we've seen include improved well-being, not all the time but commonly, and improved libido.

Edmund Chein, M.D., Palm Springs, CA.

I have not seen side effects when the DHEA is replaced in the physiological range. Too high levels can cause acne.

Ward Dean, M.D., Pensacola, FL.

On higher dosages there is facial hair in women and a deepening of voice. When the dosages are reduced, this goes away.

Barry Elson, M.D., Northampton, MA.

On the low doses that I use, such as 5 to 20 mg, I haven't noticed any side effects.

Alan Gaby, M.D., Editor, *Nutrition and Healing* newsletter.

Higher dosages may, in a minority of cases, lead to irritability, insomnia, and overstimulation. It's very uncommon to have hair growth. Acne is possible in large doses. My caution to users is not to take too much of this steroid.

Allen Green, M.D., Newport Beach, CA.

I've treated over 100 patients with DHEA and there have been no side effects except for mild acne in a small percentage of women. Most people either feel no effect from the DHEA or have a positive reaction.

Ron Hoffman, M.D., New York City, NY.

Side effects are rare and mild. I haven't seen any acne or male pattern baldness on low doses.

Michael Janson, M.D., Barnstable, MA.

I've been using DHEA for the past two years mostly as hormone replacement therapy in older adults. Having now treated more than 100 people, I have hardly seen any side effects, except perhaps for rare cases of jitteriness and insomnia. I try to keep my doses low, such as 25 mg or less.

As far as positive effects, I would say improved mood and energy are the two most mentioned. However, the majority of users do not notice an effect one way or the other.

Davis Lamson, N.D., Kent, WA.

A small percentage of women may have a skin outbreak on their scalp or face and a possible overgrowth of hair on their chin or lip. I have not noticed acne in men.

Moreover, there's a theoretical risk for breast or prostate tumor stimulation by DHEA. Therefore, a mammogram in women and PSA (prostatic surface antigen) test in men is appropriate.

Dr. Bob Martin, Phoenix, AZ.

I have not had side effects reported yet. Some patients don't feel any effect.

Gary Ross, M.D., San Francisco, CA.

There are some side effects, but they are minor. A very small percentage may have heart palpitations. In women, when the dose is too high, they may on occasion have a little acne on their face or chest. This does not occur on doses less than 15 mg.

Gerald Sugarman, M.D., Director of Lifetime Wellness in Arroyo Grande, CA.

Rarely acne, otherwise no side effects.

Jonathan V. Wright, M.D., Kent, WA.

Acne can occur in females, especially on high doses. Whiskers can crop up and there can be deepening of voice; again these are un common with physiologic replacement. Sometimes there is breast tenderness but the majority of women have no breast trouble, no lipid changes, or changes in blood glucose levels. It's important to do follow up tests regularly and check not only DHEA, but other androgens and estrogens.

Rare individuals can be to sensitive to DHEA and have hives or feel worse. A quarter of the users say they don't feel any effect.

References:

Aizawa H, Niimura M. *Adrenal androgen abnormalities in women with late onset and persistent acne.* Arch Dermatol Res 284 (8): 451-5, 1993. See also **Aizawa H**, Nakada Y, Niimura M. *Androgen status in adolescent women with acne vulgaris.* J Dermatology 22(7):530-2, 1995.

Ebeling P, Kolvisto V. *Physiological importance of DHEA.* The Lancet 343:1479-1481, 1994.

McIntosh M, Goldfarb A, Curtis L, Cote P. *Vitamin E alters hepatic antioxidant enzymes in rats treated with DHEA.* J Nutr 123 (2): 216-24, 1993.

Orner GA. *DHEA is a complete hepatocarcinogen and potent tumor promoter in the absence of peroxisome proliferation in rainbow trout.* Carcinogenesis 16:2893-95, 1995.

Rao M, Musunuri S, Reddy J. Pathobiology 60:82-86, 1992.

van Vollenhoven RF, Engleman EG, McGuire JL. *An open study of DHEA in SLE.* Arthritis Rheum 37 (9):1305-10, 1994.

Walton S, Cunliffe W. *Clinical, ultrasound and hormonal markers of androgenicity in acne vulgaris.* Br J Dermatol 133(2):249-53, 1995.

Appendix A

Everything You Always Wanted To Know About The Adrenal Glands

The two adrenal glands are triangular shaped and located above each kidney (see figures in chapter 1). *Ad*, in Latin, signifies nearness to; *renal* means of the kidneys.

The center of the adrenal gland is called the medulla (meaning marrow in Latin) and the outer covering is called the cortex (meaning bark of a tree in Latin). You may remember that our brain also has an outer layer, called the cerebral cortex.

The medulla is mostly responsible for making and secreting two chemicals known as epinephrine (the trademark name is Adrenalin) and norepinephrine. These are strong stimulants that increase heart rate and blood pressure, and make you feel nervous when too much of them are released– such as when you get up to give a speech, you search all your pockets, and you can't find your notes.

The adrenal cortex has long been known to consist of three layers, each with a different function (Hornsby, 1995).

The outermost layer is called the zona glomerulosa. It releases aldosterone, a hormone that acts on the kidneys to save sodium from the urine and excrete potassium. The zona glomerulosa releases aldosterone when it is stimulated by another hormone called angiotensin. The liver is the organ responsible for releasing angiotensinogen, the precursor to angiotensin. Recently it has been found that *ACTH* (adrenocorticotrophic hormone), a hormone released by the pituitary gland, also stimulates aldosterone production (Daidoh, 1995). Aldosterone generally has a blood pressure raising effect since it helps the kidneys save sodium. As you know, sodium, a component of salt, raises blood pressure.

The middle layer of the adrenal cortex is called the zona fasciculata. This layer produces and secretes glucocorticoids, the best known one being cortisol, a very powerful hormone that has anti-inflammatory effects. The zona fasciculata releases glucocorticoids when stimulated by ACTH. ACTH is released more often during times of stress.

The inner layer is called the zona reticularis. This layer is primarily responsible for making the hormones DHEA and DHEAS. ACTH, and possibly other factors, also stimulate the production of DHEA.

ACTH (from pituitary gland) and angiotensin (from liver) ⟶ *zona glomerulosa* ⟶ **Aldosterone**

ACTH (from pituitary gland) ⟶ *zona fasciculata* ⟶ **Cortisol and other glucocorticoids**

ACTH (from pituitary gland) and possibly other factors ⟶ *zona reticularis* ⟶ **DHEA, DHEAS, androgens** and **estrogens**

At least 150 steroids are produced either by the adrenal cortex or by metabolism of these steroids elsewhere in the body (Murphy, 1993). Some of the best-known of these steroids are cortisol, testosterone, DHEA(S), and estrogen. The level of DHEAS in serum is about 10 times that of cortisol.

Each of the steroids mentioned above undergoes extensive metabolism resulting in 20 or more metabolites. When DHEA and DHEAS travel to our tissues and enter our cells, they are changed into androgens, estrogens, and other steroids. Numerous enzymes are present in our cells that are involved in this metabolism: 5-alpha-reductase, aromatase, sulfotransferase, 17-beta-hydroxysteriod dehydrogenase, etc. As we age, the activity of these enzymes is altered.

The conversion of hormones to other metabolites within our

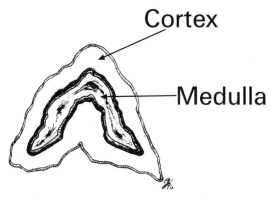

Cross-Section of Adrenal Gland

cells has been termed "Intracrinology" (Labrie, 1991). The conversion of these hormones to other steroids within our cells makes it difficult for us to know the specific hormonal status of our tissues when based solely on blood samples.

It is interesting to note that ACTH influences the release of aldosterone, cortisol, and DHEA. Cortisol levels stay approximately the same throughout life, but DHEA(S) levels drop. Therefore, there may be changes going on within the adrenal glands that lead to the decline in DHEA(S) (Belanger, 1994). These changes are not yet fully understood.

References:

Daidoh H, Morita H, Mune T, Murayama M, Hanafusa J, Ni H. *Responses of plasma adrenocortical steroids to low dose ACTH in normal subjects.* Clin Endocrinol (Oxf) 43(3):311-5, 1995. As low a dose as 0.1 mcg of ACTH stimulated aldosterone release while 0.5 mcg was needed for cortisol and DHEA release. This leads us to wonder whether even low levels of stress, by releasing ACTH from the pituitary, can increase blood pressure through effects by aldosterone on salt retention.

Hornsby P. *Biosynthesis of DHEAS by the human adrenal cortex and its age-related decline.* Ann NY Acad Sci 774:29-46, 1995.

Labrie F. *Intracrinology.* Mol Cell Endocrinol 78:C113-118, 1991.

Murphy B, Wolkowitz O. *The pathophysiologic significance of hyperadrenocorticism: antiglucocorticoid strategies.* Psychiatric Annals 23:12, 1993.

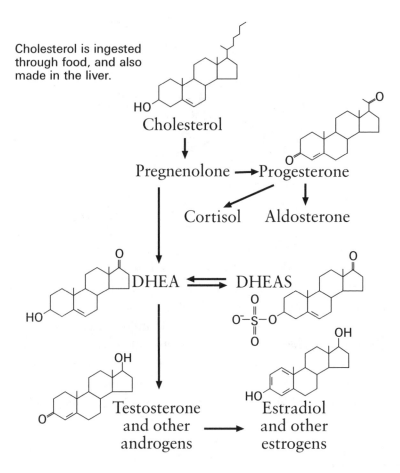

Cholesterol is ingested
through food, and also
made in the liver.

Cholesterol

Pregnenolone ⟶ Progesterone

Cortisol   Aldosterone

DHEA ⇌ DHEAS

Testosterone
and other
androgens

⟶

Estradiol
and other
estrogens

*Please note that some
metabolic steps have been skipped
in order to simplify this diagram*

Metabolism of Cholesterol
in the Adrenal Glands to
DHEA and Other Steroids

THE DEA AND THE FDA AND THE DSHEA ON DHEA

D
HEA has been available by prescription from compounding pharmacies for more than ten years. The practice of compounding involves the formulation of custom medications for patients with particular needs. As this practice predates the passage of the 1938 Food Drug & Cosmetic Act, these pharmacies have a lot of latitude to formulate medicines that would otherwise not be easily available. For the past decade, a few doctors had been prescribing DHEA to their patients who then obtained this steroid through these pharmacies. But the need for a prescription ended with the passage of a new law.

In November of 1994, after an arduous legal battle, a new law was passed by Congress called the Dietary Supplement Health & Education Act (DSHEA). For the first time in its history, Congress defined dietary supplements as vitamins, minerals, amino acids, other dietary constituents, and herbs (and concentrates, extracts and derivatives of the above). More importantly, dietary supplements were to be considered foods, not drugs. The FDA regards a drug as any medicine that "alters the structure or function of the human body" or is intended to "treat, prevent, cure, or mitigate a disease."

An example of a supplement that is now more readily available for sale in the US as a consequence of the passage of the DSHEA law is the hormone melatonin, a derivative of the amino acid tryptophan. In order for the FDA to challenge melatonin's over-the-counter status, it has to prove that this hormone is not safe. Since the passage of DSHEA, the burden of proof for a

substance not being safe now rests on the FDA, not the producers
or retailers. This shift has both positive and negative consequences
for the consumer. A wider selection of supplements are now on
the shelves of the health food stores or through mail order firms,
but less of a guarantee that these have been thoroughly evaluated before being marketed. The consumer now has to make an
even greater attempt to self-educate before casually swallowing
the newest pills on the market.

The DSHEA on DHEA

With the new law in place, what is the legal status of DHEA? A
drug because it "alters the structure or function of the human
body" or because it is intended to "treat, prevent, cure or mitigate
a disease"? A drug can be regulated by the FDA. Or is DHEA a
dietary supplement because it is a derivative of cholesterol, which
is itself a constituent of food, and not under the FDA's jurisdic-
tion? As you can see, arguments can be made for both sides.

The DEA on DHEA

As DHEA started entering the over-the-counter US supplement
market, there were hints that the Drug Enforcement Agency
(DEA) was considering classifying it as an anabolic steroid. The
Controlled Substances Act requires that any substance that is
structurally related to testosterone and has testosterone-like
anabolic properties be scheduled as an anabolic steroid. DHEA
is a precursor to testosterone, and so it has a structural similarity
to testosterone. But so is cholesterol; it is also a precursor, and
structurally related, to both DHEA and testosterone.

The DEA eventually chose not to pursue any plans to schedule
DHEA as a controlled substance.

The FDA on DHEA

For now the FDA seems to have taken a laissez-faire attitude with
DHEA by not interfering with its over-the-counter sale. Will it
continue to keep its distance as the popularity of DHEA
increases? Or when promoters of this steroid continue making
outlandish, "fountain of youth," claims? Time will tell.

What do you think of DHEA being available without a prescription?

Etienne-Emile Baulieu, M.D., Ph.D., Director, Department of Hormone Research of the Institut National de la Sante et de la Recherche Medicale, Paris, France.

DHEA and DHEAS are not toxic, in the sense that we all live normally with these steroids circulating in the blood (and in very high concentrations for DHEAS). Studies in laboratory animals are not directly relevant since they do not have significant concentrations of DHEA and DHEAS in the blood, contrary to higher primates. However, in humans, as well as in animals, DHEA and DHEAS can be transformed into active sex steroids, such as testosterone, 5-alpha-dihydrotestosterone and estrogens, particularly but not exclusively in the liver, and these sex steroids have their own targets with well-known physiological and pathological consequences. Practically, low doses of administered DHEA leading to concentrations of DHEAS in the range of young people do not lead to a significant increase of sex steroids in the blood. What would be risky is that people take daily a large dose, leading to an excess of circulating active sex steroids.

I advise people to take it only under the guidance of a physician. Further studies may provide more liberal conclusions, but for the time being, I am against its over-the-counter sale.

Michael Bennett, M.D., Department of Pathology, University of Texas Southwestern Medical Center in Dallas.

As long as it is sold in low doses such as 25 mg, I see no problems with it. DHEA is not toxic at this level. Humans have been given up to 1,600 mg without problems. Since this steroid is not patentable, drug companies are not going to make the effort to research all its potential benefits and make it available to the public. Therefore, if vitamin companies don't sell them, chances are few other sources will. What is needed is an effort by the food industry to conduct research with low doses of DHEA.

Peter Hornsby, Ph.D., Huffington Center on Aging, Baylor College of Medicine, Houston, TX.

It's terrible that consumers can buy it without a prescription. The clinical trials are only in their infancy. We know a lot about what DHEA does in rodents but have little clue about the long-term effects in humans. It could perhaps be disastrous. DHEA has an androgenic effect on women which could cause negative changes in their lipid profile (cholesterol, triglycerides). Whether this could increase their risk for heart disease is not clear.

Christopher Longcope, Ph.D., Department of Obstetrics and Gynecology, University of Massachusetts Medical School, Worcester.

It's a natural human hormone and it's not toxic. I have no problems with it. People should have the choice if they want to use it.

Ron von Vollenhoven, M.D., Ph.D., Division of Immunology and Rheumatology, Stanford University Medical Center, CA.

I have mixed feelings. There are a number of people that may benefit from it, but I have concerns about the purity when its sold without being regulated.

Owen Wolkowitz, M.D., Department of Psychiatry at the University of California, San Francisco.

This steroid appears benign and I doubt that it would be harmful in physiologic replacement doses, but more research needs to be done, especially with long-term treatment.

Roy Walford, M.D., a leader in anti-aging research, is a professor at the University of California, Los Angeles.

I have no problems with DHEA being available to the public without a prescription since people need to have the freedom to self-experiment.

This steroid is probably innocuous, there are few adverse effects that I know of. However, the beneficial effects on the rate of aging are not yet established.

Clinicians:

Edmund Chein, M.D., Palm Springs, CA.

DHEA being available without a prescription can be dangerous, especially in men since if they take it in high doses without having their levels monitored it could increase testosterone levels and promote the growth of prostatic cancer cells. The FDA should not allow DHEA to be sold without a prescription.

Ward Dean, M.D., Pensacola, FL.

Along with the availability of melatonin, it is a major breakthrough in giving individuals the opportunity to use a supplement for life extension purposes.

Dale Guyer, M.D., Indianapolis, IN.

With DHEA, more is not necessarily better. I feel uncomfortable with people buying 25 mg or 50 mg over the counter and self-dosing. If DHEA were available without a prescription in only 5 mg or 10 mg doses, I wouldn't have any problems with that.

Davis Lamson, N.D., Kent, WA.

This steroid has broad biological functions. I don't think it should be available over the counter since many users are not discriminating enough. They'll believe whatever they read in hypish articles. A doctor's supervision is essential.

Dr. Bob Martin, Phoenix, AZ.

I'm hesitant about it being available over the counter since there may be people who might abuse it such as teenagers using it for anabolic reasons.

Gary Ross, M.D., San Francisco, CA.

I have mixed feelings. It would be wiser if DHEA were prescribed by someone with clinical experience. However, I also feel people should have the right to self-medicate. The drawback is that some people are very gullible and may buy into the hype surrounding not only DHEA, but other nutrients and products. I would certainly recommend, even if people buy it over the counter, to see a physician and get a blood test. If the levels of DHEA are low, then they can start at a low dose such as 5 or 10 mg.

Jonathan V. Wright, M.D., Kent, WA.

I can see it both ways. On one hand, I strongly believe that in an ideal society with everyone being well-educated, we should be as free as possible to purchase almost any medicine that we want to over the counter, except for hard narcotics. On the other hand, I realize that some people are not going to be informed enough when making the decision to use substances such as hormones that can influence their body in many ways. It's a tough call.

And now, the author's opinion:

I take the fifth.

No, I changed my mind. I'll voice my 2 cents' worth.

As some researchers have stated, DHEA is not toxic in low doses. The long-term consequences of high-dose use are not fully known since we understand so little about this steroid and how it metabolizes into estrogens, androgens, and other hormones. However, I believe as a culture that we need to be consistent in our approach with any supplement, food, or substance. If we were to make everything that could potentially harm us illegal, then certainly tobacco, alcohol, aspirin, and acetaminophen (Tylenol) would have to go. Aspirin can cause stomach ulcers and bleeding; regular acetominophen use can cause liver and kidney damage. Both can be fatal in overdose. And if we took things to an extreme, we might even have to ration high-fat ice cream, candy, and certain fast food chain visits.

Based on everything that has been published about DHEA, and my interviews with researchers and experienced clinicians, I believe a good compromise would be to have this steroid available to the consumer in 5 or 10 mg strengths. Heavy emphasis would have to be placed on recommending a physician's supervision while supplementing. It would be even better if the FDA or certain consumer groups occasionally spot tested the different products on the market to make sure the labeling was accurate.

Appendix C

Personal Stories of DHEA Users

I started with 25 mg a day, and in three weeks time, I noticed improved libido.

BD, Psychiatrist, male, 53, Marina del Rey, CA

For the past year I have been taking 25 mg of DHEA prescribed to me by my physician. I have heard people can live longer for taking it and their immune system can improve. This has been enough of an incentive for me to keep using it. I have not noticed any influence on libido or motivation, nor have I noticed any side effects. Perhaps I'm not as much of a type A person as I used to be.

LB, 53, male, writer and inventor, Hollywood, CA

Since beginning to take DHEA at 50 mg a day, I have noticed a marked increase in my libido. I'm a 43 year old male and I find myself as horny as I was at 17, having sex two or three times a day and enjoying it more than I have in years. I wonder how common a reaction this is to DHEA. I assume this is because of an increase in testosterone levels due to conversion of DHEA— is there any danger of downregulating my natural testosterone production if I continue to take DHEA at this dosage? I sure hope not, because I am **really** having a good time. In fact, this is so much fun that I am sure it won't be too much longer before the government makes it illegal.

Posted on the internet in sci.life-extension newsgroup

For the past year I've been taking 100 mg of DHEA every day. To be honest, I have noticed absolutely nothing. My wife has been taking 100 mg every other day. She also has noticed nothing. We both take it with the hopes of living longer.

LS, 53, Los Angeles, CA

I read in *Time* magazine the research done by Dr. Yen where he found positive effects of DHEA supplementation. In July of 1995, I started using DHEA at 50 mg at night. A few weeks later I noticed my sexual performance to be improved– back to being a 30 year old. I'm also in a better mood and more relaxed. There have been no side effects. I was hoping my arthritis would get better but I've seen little help with my aches and pains. I'm not sure but maybe I have more muscle mass.

HW, 68, Los Angeles

I started DHEA at 50 mg two weeks ago and I haven't seen any effects yet.

WM, Ph.D., 46, male

I've been off my estrogen replacement therapy for the past 2 months and a week ago I started 25 mg DHEA every other day. Soon afterwards I noticed a small blemish on my face and a slight decrease in appetite. However, my energy level seems to have been boosted and I feel flirtatious. I'm planning to go back on estrogen, in addition to the DHEA.

Barbara Perlman, 52, Marina Del Rey, CA

I have been taking 30 mg daily after breakfast (to slow absorption and to minimize conflict with melatonin taken at night). I am 47 and very active and I definitely feel better and stronger for that DHEA capsule. I can't quantify it any better than that because it is quite an intangible improvement. I have definitely noticed an increase in libido which makes me worried about increasing my dosage.

GC, FL

For the last four months I've been taking 50 mg of micronized DHEA. Before I started, my blood levels were normal for my age, but low compared to youth levels. I've noticed more energy, the ability to tolerate longer workouts at the gym, and certainly more dreams. My libido hasn't improved, then again, it really didn't need to. Older physicians with whom I work have told me that they have noticed their libido to increase after starting DHEA.

On the downside, I'm not sure if my male pattern baldness is progressing faster since starting the DHEA. I plan to continue taking this steroid for its possible long-term health benefits but I intend to lower the dose.

Gary Randall, Ph.D., HCLD, 43, Andrologist, Columbia Indian Path Medical Center, Kingsport, TN

I'm a 46 year old woman and for the past 8 months I've been taking 12.5 mg of DHEA twice a day. I now have more stamina and my libido has improved. I feel 30 again.

PL, Topanga, CA

My doctor has me on 25 mg of DHEA since my blood levels were low. In addition to the DHEA, I'm also on natural progesterone cream. I can't take estrogen because of uterine fibroids.

When I was placed on 50 mg a day, I had too high testosterone levels and my doctor reduced my dose to 25 mg. Since being on it, I feel more flexible and find my body doesn't ache anymore when I get out of bed. I also feel more energized and have noticed increased libido.

Miki Herman, 51, Sherman Oaks, CA

GLOSSARY

Acetylcholine– a chemical found in the nervous system and used to transmit nerve impulses. In the brain, acetylcholine is involved with memory.

ACTH (adrenocorticotrophic hormone)– a hormone secreted by the pituitary gland. It stimulates the adrenal gland to make steroids.

Albumin– a class of proteins found in milk, eggs, muscle tissue and blood. They can be broken down into amino acids.

Aldosterone– a steroid hormone produced by the adrenal cortex, where its major function is to facilitate potassium exchange for sodium in the kidney, causing sodium reabsorption and potassium excretion. This leads to the raising of blood pressure.

Alzheimer's disease– A progressive brain disease leading to memory loss, interference with thinking abilities, and other losses of mental powers. Brain cells show degenerative damage.

Amino acid– a molecule that serves as a unit of structure of proteins and contains nitrogen. Twenty-two amino acids are found in the human body, including arginine, lysine, tryptophan, and phenylalanine. Eight out of the 22 are essential, that is, the body cannot make them. These need to be ingested through foods.

Androgen– a hormone that encourages the development of male sexual characteristics. Some of the androgens made by the adrenal glands are DHEA, DHEAS, androstenedione, and testosterone.

Angiotensin– a substance made of ten amino acids that has the ability to constrict blood vessels and stimulate aldosterone release. Angiotensinogen, a substance formed by the liver and present in the blood, is converted by the enzyme renin into angiotensin. Renin is released by the kidneys.

Antibody– a protein produced in response to contact of the body with an antigen. It has the specific capacity of neutralizing an antigen.

Antigen– a substance, bacteria, virus, or toxin to which the body reacts by forming antibodies.

Antioxidant– a substance that combines with damaging molecules, neutralizes them, and thus prevents the deterioration of DNA, RNA, lipids, and proteins. Vitamins C, E, and beta carotene are the best-known antioxidants, but more and more are being discovered each year. It is believed that one aspect of aging is the slow degeneration and breakdown of chemicals within our cells. Antioxidants are thought to prevent or slow down this degenerative process.

Autoimmune– immunity against self. The body makes antibodies that attack and damage its own cells. Systemic lupus erythematosus is one such condition.

Benzodiazepine– a class of medicines such as Valium , Dalmane, and Restoril that act on GABA receptors to induce relaxation and sleep. Too much, used too often, can lead to memory loss.

Cell membrane– a thin layer consisting mostly of fatty acids that forms the lining of each cell.

Cholesterol– the most abundant steroid in animal tissues. It is present in some of the foods we eat. Our liver can also make some if there's not enough in our diet.

Control– in many studies, whenever a group of animals or humans are given a certain medicine, they are compared to another group of animals or humans who are in under the same circumstances for everything except the medicine. This second group is known as the controls. This way, researchers can find out what the role of the medicine was independent of any other factors.

Coronary– There are two arteries that supply blood to our heart, the left and the right coronaries. A heart attack occurs when one of these arteries, or a smaller offshoot, becomes blocked, either by a blood clot (coronary thrombosis), or by plaque. Small doses of blood thinners, such as aspirin, are thought to reduce the rate of heart attacks by decreasing blood clotting by platelets. A coronary can also mean "heart attack."

Cortisol– a sterol (related to steroid) secreted by the human adrenal glands. High doses lead to interference with the proper functioning of the immune system.

Cytomegalovirus– a type of virus that can invade cells of many organs, but especially the salivary glands. A person with a normal immunity generally would not succumb to this virus.

Diosgenin– a sapogenin derived from the saponins discin and trillin found in the roots of plants such as the yam. In the laboratory, parts of this molecule can be cleaved in order to make certain steroids. The steroid portion, 5-spirostene, serves as a source from which pregnenolone and progesterone can be prepared. Our body is not known to have the proper enzymes to convert diosgenin into pregnenolone, progesterone or DHEA. Therefore, ingesting wild yam extracts will not lead to DHEA production.

Epinephrine– a hormone made by the medulla of the adrenal gland and also made in the brain and other parts of the nervous system. The product name is Adrenalin. It is a potent stimulator of heart rate, tightens some blood vessels, relaxes others, and relaxes the bronchi (tubes) in the lungs. In the brain it is considered a neurotransmitter that leads to alertness and vigilance. Epinephrine is made by the amino acids phenylalanine and tyrosine.

Estrogen– a hormone made by the ovaries, adrenal glands, and also in various cells of the body. Estrogen promotes female characteristics. The most common estrogens are estrone, estradiol, and estriol. Premarin, a product name for conjugated estrogens, is actually derived from the urine of horses.

GABA– gamma amino butyric acid, a brain chemical that causes sedation. Medicines such as Valium act on receptors for GABA to induce relaxation.

Glucocorticoid– any steroid-like compound capable of significantly influencing some aspects of metabolism, such as the promotion of glycogen deposition in the liver, and having anti-inflammatory effects. Cortisol is the most potent of the naturally occurring glucocorticoids, but some synthetic derivatives, such as prednisone, are more potent.

Gonad– a testicle or ovary.

Hormone– a chemical messenger produced by a gland or organ that influences a number of metabolic actions in our cells. Some hormones have been studied for a number of years, such as estrogen, which has been given to women after menopause for over 20 years.

Hypothalamus– a small area of the brain above and behind the roof of the mouth. The hypothalamus is prominently involved with the functions of the autonomic nervous system and the hormonal system. It also plays a role in mood and motivation.

Immune globulins– a group of proteins found in blood. Immune globulins (or immunoglobulins) fight off infections by attaching to and killing bacteria and viruses. The best known is gamma globulin.

Insulin– a hormone made by the pancreas that helps regulate blood sugar levels.

Interferon– a small protein produced by white blood cells to fight infections, especially viral, and some forms of cancer.

Interleukin– similar to interferon, a small protein produced by white blood cells to fight infections and some forms of cancer. There are many types of interleukins, numbered 1, 2, 3, up to 10 or more. Some interleukins are beneficial, while others may have negative effects on the immune system.

Leukemia– a cancer of white blood cells that results in their abnormal growth and multiplication. Leukemias can have a slow onset and progression, called *chronic*, or a sudden onset, called *acute*.

Libido– sex drive.

Lymphocyte– a type of white blood cell. Two major types are B lymphocytes and T lymphocytes.

Lymphokine– a substance released by lymphocytes to help with immune function. Interferon is a type of lymphokine.

Lymphoma– any of a group of diseases characterized by painless, progressive enlargement of lymph glands. Hodgkin's disease is a form of lymphoma.

Macrophage– a large cell of the immune system that has the ability to be phagocytic, that is, engulf and kill germs. This cell is also thought to be involved in plaque formation in arteries.

Metabolism– the chemical and physical processes continuously going in the body involving the creation and breakdown of molecules.

Molecule– the smallest possible quantity of atoms that retains the chemical properties of the substance. For instance, a molecule of water consists of three atoms, two hydrogen and one oxygen.

Monocyte– A large white blood cell normally found in lymphoid tissues such as spleen, bone marrow, and lymph nodes.

Multiple Sclerosis– a chronic disease in which there is loss of myelin (the covering of a nerve) of the central nervous system. It is characterized by speech defects and loss of muscular coordination.

Mycobacteria– Mycobacterium is the singular; a type of bacterium within the same genus as the ones that cause tuberculosis and leprosy. It has the shape of a rod and is Gram positive.

Natural killer cell– a type of white blood cell that can destroy certain cancer cells and germs.

Neuron– a brain cell. There are over 100 billion of these cells in our brain. Neurons communicate with each other through chemicals called neurotransmitters.

Neurotransmitter– a biochemical substance, such as norepinephrine, serotonin, dopamine, phenylethylamine, acetylcholine, and endorphin, that relays messages from one neuron to another.

NMDA (not to be confused with the popular street drug MDMA, a.k.a. 'Ecstasy')– a type of receptor on our neurons (brain cells). It stands for N-methyl-D-aspartate. This receptor plays an important role in regulating the function and form of synapses on our neurons thus influencing learning and memory. Aging is thought to be associated with a decline in the number of NMDA receptors, which may partly account for loss of learning ability and memory in old age. Interestingly, the administration of acetyl-l-carnitine (a nutrient and antioxidant found in vitamin stores) slows the age-associated reduction in the number of these receptors in rodents (Castorina M, et al. *A cluster analysis study of acetyl-l-carnitine effect on NMDA receptors in aging.* Experimental Gerontology 28:537-548, 1993.)

Norepinephrine– a hormone made by the adrenal medulla. It is similar in some ways to epinephrine but weaker.

Peroxisome– an organelle (small organ or structure) occurring in animal and plant cells that has enzymes relating to the formation and degradation of cholesterol, prostaglandins, and fatty acids. Peroxisomes are also involved in antioxidant activities.

Placebo– a dummy pill that contains no active ingredient.

Platelet– a small, round or oval cell found in the blood involved in blood clotting.

Pneumococcus– a bacterium that is a causative agent of pneumonia and of certain other diseases. Vaccines for different strains are available.

Precursor– a substance that is the source of another substance.

Pregnenolone– the steroid from which most other steroids are formed, including DHEA. See Appendix A for the chemistry.

Prostate gland– a partly muscular gland surrounding the urethra at the base of the bladder. It secretes a lubricating fluid that is discharged with the sperm. Enlargement of this gland is known as BPH, benign prostatic hypertrophy.

Receptor– a special arrangement on a cell that recognizes a molecule and interacts with it. This allows the molecule to either enter the cell or stimulate it in a specific way.

Renin– an enzyme made by the kidneys that breaks down angiotensinogen into angiotensin.

Sebaceous gland– a gland in the skin that usually opens into the hair follicles and secretes an oily, semifluid substance known as sebum.

Serotonin– a brain chemical (neurotransmitter) that relays messages between brain cells (neurons). It is one of the primary mood neurotransmitters. It is derived form the amino acid tryptophan. Serotonin can also be converted to melatonin.

Sterol– a steroid of 27 or more carbon atoms with one OH (alcohol) group. Cholesterol is a sterol.

Testosterone– a hormone made by the testicles and adrenal glands, and also in various cells of the body, that promotes masculine traits.

Thymus– a gland located in the upper part of the chest. It is involved in the development of the immune system, especially the maturation of T lymphocytes.

Triglyceride– a type of fat that circulates in the bloodstream. A glycerol molecule forms the backbone to which 1, 2, or 3 fatty acids attach. High blood triglyceride levels can lead to atherosclerosis (blockage of arteries).

INDEX

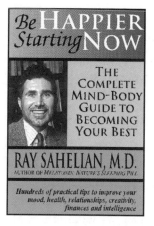

A self-actualization book unlike any in its genre. In addressing one of the most universal of human quests— happiness— it promotes a humanist approach. The mind-body connection is explained in terms of interactions of the neural, hormonal, and immune systems.

Skeptical Enquirer, July/August, 1995

I know the literature on melatonin quite well since I have done a great deal of research on it. Thus, I was pleasantly surprised at how accurate your book is and how useful it will be for patients, professionals, and researchers alike. I passed your book on to some of my colleagues and they were all very impressed!

James Jan, M.D., melatonin researcher, British Columbia's Children's Hospital, Vancouver, Canada

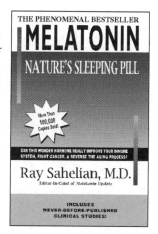

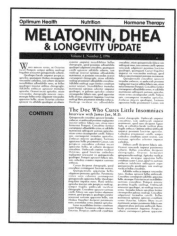

Would you like to keep up to date with the latest research? *Melatonin, DHEA and Longevity Update* is a newsletter that can be a reliable source for you. You don't have to read hundreds of detailed scientific articles. We'll summarize, translate, and interpret the latest findings for you.

Each issue has interviews with top researchers across the globe. Breakthrough nutritional studies on longevity will also be discussed. The first issue was published in January, 1996.

I would like:

❑ To be placed on your mailing list for information about future books, upcoming lectures and seminars in my area, or any other related information. (*free*)

❑ Information about physicians in my area who are familiar with DHEA (*please send a self-addressed stamped envelope*)

Name: _____

Address: _____

City/State/Zip: _____

Phone: _____

❑ I am a health care professional. Please add me to your directory. My specialty is: _____

I am sending a check. I would like:

___ copies *Melatonin: Nature's Sleeping Pill* $13.95   _____

___ copies *Be Happier Starting Now* $12.00   _____

___ copies *DHEA: A Practical Guide* $ 9.95   _____

❑ 4 issues of *Melatonin, DHEA & Longevity Update* $16.00   _____

❑ 8 issues of *Melatonin, DHEA & Longevity Update* $28.00   _____

❑ 16 issues of *Melatonin, DHEA & Longevity Update* $48.00   _____

No shipping charge for the books if mailed to a US or Canadian destination.

Shipping for overseas mailings, add $5 per book or 50¢ per newsletter _____

Tax on books mailed to California residents is 8%.   _____

                                                         Total $ _____

Discounts available for multiple copies. Call for details.

Books and newsletters are shipped promptly. Indicate if you would like your book to be personally autographed by Dr. Sahelian.

Please send a check for the full amount to the following address:

      Be Happier Press
      PO Box 12619
      Marina Del Rey, CA 90295
      T: 310-821-2409

You may also order by credit card, either by phone or mail. Visa, MC, AE, Diner's Club, Carte Blanche, and JCB cards accepted. If by mail, include your current account number and expiration date.

Best times to phone are weekdays between 9 am and 5 pm (Pacific time).

Be Happier Press
P. O. Box 12619
Marina Del Rey, CA 90295

Be Happier Press
P. O. Box 12619
Marina Del Rey, CA 90295

I would like:

❏ To be placed on your mailing list for information about future books, upcoming lectures and seminars in my area, or any other related information. *(free)*

❏ Information about physicians in my area who are familiar with DHEA *(please send a self-addressed stamped envelope)*

Name: _____

Address: _____

City/State/Zip: _____

Phone: _____

❏ I am a health care professional. Please add me to your directory. My specialty is: _____

I am sending a check. I would like:

___ copies *Melatonin: Nature's Sleeping Pill*	$13.95	_____
___ copies *Be Happier Starting Now*	$12.00	_____
___ copies *DHEA: A Practical Guide*	$ 9.95	_____
❏ 4 issues of *Melatonin, DHEA & Longevity Update*	$16.00	_____
❏ 8 issues of *Melatonin, DHEA & Longevity Update*	$28.00	_____
❏ 16 issues of *Melatonin, DHEA & Longevity Update*	$48.00	_____

No shipping charge for the books if mailed to a US or Canadian destination.

Shipping for overseas mailings, add $5 per book or 50¢ per newsletter _____

Tax on books mailed to California residents is 8%. _____

Total $ _____

Discounts available for multiple copies. Call for details.

Books and newsletters are shipped promptly. Indicate if you would like your book to be personally autographed by Dr. Sahelian.

Please send a check for the full amount to the following address:

Be Happier Press
PO Box 12619
Marina Del Rey, CA 90295
T: 310-821-2409

You may also order by credit card, either by phone or mail. Visa, MC, AE, Diner's Club, Carte Blanche, and JCB cards accepted. If by mail, include your current account number and expiration date.

Best times to phone are weekdays between 9 am and 5 pm (Pacific time).